Responsibilisation at the Margins of Welfare Services

T0298663

The impetus for this book is the shift in welfare policy in Western Europe from state responsibilities to individual and community responsibilities. The book examines the ways in which policies associated with advanced liberalism and New Public Management can be identified as influencing professional practices to promote personalisation, participation, empowerment, recovery and resilience. In examining the concept of 'responsibilisation' from the point of view of both the 'responsibilised client and welfare worker', the book breaks from the traditional literature to demonstrate how responsibilities are negotiated during multi-professional care planning meetings, home visits, staff meetings, focus groups and interviews with different stakeholders.

The settings examined in the book can be described as on the 'margins of welfare' – mental health, substance abuse, homelessness services and probation work, where the rights and responsibilities of clients and workers are uncertain and constantly under review. Each chapter approaches the management of responsibilities from a particular angle by combining responsibilisation theory and discourse analysis to examine everyday encounters. Taken together, the chapters paint a comprehensive picture of the responsibilisation practices at the margins of welfare services and provide an extensive discussion of the implications for policy and practice.

Drawing upon both the governmentality literature and everyday encounters, the book provides a broad approach to a key topic. It will therefore be a valuable resource for social policy, public administration, social work and human service researchers and students, and social and health care professionals.

Kirsi Juhila is Professor in social work in the School of Social Sciences and Humanities at the University of Tampere, Finland.

Suvi Raitakari is Senior Lecturer in social work in the School of Social Sciences and Humanities at the University of Tampere, Finland.

Christopher Hall is Visiting Senior Research Fellow in the Department of Social Work and Social Care at the University of Sussex, UK.

Routledge Advances in Social Work

Responsibilisation at the Margins of Welfare Services

Edited by Kirsi Juhila,
Suvi Raitakari and
Christopher Hall

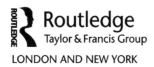

Routledge
Taylor & Francis Group

LONDON AND NEW YORK

First published 2017 by Routledge

2 Park Square, Milton Park, Abingdon, Oxon OX14 4RN
605 Third Avenue, New York, NY 10017

Routledge is an imprint of the Taylor & Francis Group, an informa business

First issued in paperback 2021

British Library Cataloguing in Publication Data
A catalogue record for this book is available from the British Library

Library of Congress Cataloging in Publication Data
Names: Juhila, Kirsi, editor. | Raitakari, Suvi, editor. |
Hall, Christopher, 1948- editor.
Title: Responsibilization at the margins of welfare services / edited by Kirsi Juhila, Suvi Raitakari and Christopher Hall.
Description: Abingdon, Oxon ; New York, NY : Routledge, 2016. |
Series: Routledge advances in social work | Includes index.
Identifiers: LCCN 2016027610| ISBN 9781138928381 (hardback) |
ISBN 9781315681757 (ebook)
Subjects: LCSH: Social service–Europe. | Social service–Practice–Europe.
Social work administration–Europe. | Public welfare–Europe.
Classification: LCC HV238 .R473 2016 | DDC 361.6068–dc23
LC record available at https://lccn.loc.gov/2016027610

ISBN: 978-1-138-92838-1 (hbk)
ISBN: 978-1-138-36097-6 (pbk)

Typeset in Times New Roman
by Wearset Ltd, Boldon, Tyne and Wear

Contents

Contributors

Dorte Caswell is Associate Professor in social work and social policy in the Department of Sociology and Social Work at Aalborg University, Denmark.

Kirsi Günther is Lecturer in social work in the School of Social Sciences and Humanities at the University of Tampere, Finland.

Christopher Hall is Visiting Senior Research Fellow in the Department of Social Work and Social Care at the University of Sussex, UK.

Cecilia Hansen Löfstrand is Associate Professor in sociology in the Department of Sociology and Work Science at the University of Gothenburg, Sweden.

Kirsi Juhila is Professor in social work in the School of Social Sciences and Humanities at the University of Tampere, Finland.

Lisa Morriss is Senior Research Associate in the Department of Sociology at Lancaster University, UK.

Nichlas Permin Berger is Researcher at the Danish Institute for Local and Regional Government Research, Denmark.

Suvi Raitakari is Senior Lecturer in social work in the School of Social Sciences and Humanities at the University of Tampere, Finland.

Jenni-Mari Räsänen is Post-doctoral Researcher in social work in the School of Social Sciences and Humanities at the University of Tampere, Finland.

Sirpa Saario is Post-doctoral Researcher in social work in the School of Social Sciences and Humanities at the University of Tampere, Finland.

Acknowledgements

First of all we wish to thank the service users and the practitioners in our field sites. Without their active participation and engagement we would not have been able to produce a realistic account. The book is dedicated to them.

The funding provided by the Finnish Academy for the projects *Responsibilization of service users and professionals in mental health practices* (2011–2016) and *Long-term homelessness and Finnish adaptations of the Housing First model* (2011–2015) has enabled our focus on researching the management of responsibilities in Finland and in England. The research was conducted in the School of Social Sciences and Humanities at the University of Tampere with the partnership of the School of Medicine, Pharmacy and Health at Durham University.

In addition we wish to thank all the members of the Network of *Discourse and Narrative Approaches to Social Work and Counselling* (DANASWAC) for valuable comments and inspiration regarding the early versions of the chapters.

1 Introduction

Kirsi Juhila, Suvi Raitakari and Christopher Hall

Managing responsibilities between parties

Dave and Carol, a client and a worker in a supported housing service, sit in Carol's office with the purpose of discussing whether Dave's care plan has been actualised up to this point. Carol initiates the topic:

CAROL: You don't seem to have progressed in this housing support service as was originally agreed in your care plan. You haven't attended our group activities for a while, and you haven't always been at home when we've come to visit you. Also, you still seem to use drugs every now and then. Do you remember how three months ago we agreed, when we were completing your care plan, that you would join in with group activities and commit to an addiction rehabilitation process?

DAVE: I have tried my best. But I didn't know exactly what the plan meant back then. I just don't feel comfortable with joining group activities and talking about my life for home visit workers. I haven't been well, and sometimes I find the expectations too much. But it is really great that I've now got my own place to live, after so much homelessness.

CAROL: Good to hear that, but unfortunately we can't make any exceptions for you, Dave, since we have a contract with the council that means we have to make a certain amount of home visits each month, and to offer group activities for our clients. The contract also says you have to commit to abstinence during a rehabilitation process. I know these rules sound really inflexible, but that's how it is. Perhaps we should start working out a service and housing option that suits your wishes better, although I know it's really difficult, with the service options that are available in this city at the moment.

DAVE: Does this mean I might end up homeless again?

CAROL: We try to avoid it in every way. The next step could be to ask your social worker to arrange a care planning meeting, where we can assess your current situation and decide on your future service options with other professionals.

DAVE: Okay.

Although not an actual dialogue between a worker and client in a supported housing service setting, this exchange displays many of the key features of the management of responsibilities in services at the margins of welfare. It is typical of the dilemmas that have emerged from our multiple empirical investigations and which will be examined in this book. To begin with, Dave is expected to fulfil his responsibilities as a client: for example, to participate actively in his recovery process in ways that have been agreed in a care plan. The worker's responsibilities, on the other hand, include helping, supporting and advising the client in his recovery process, and also checking up and reminding him if he neglects or does not fulfil the agreed responsibilities. However, responsibilities are not managed only between the client and the worker, but also between the worker as a representative of a service provider and the purchaser of services (the local council). The supported housing service has a contract with the municipality that regulates the contents of service packages (e.g. home visits, group activities, commitment to abstinence during a rehabilitation process). The service provider therefore has responsibilities in two directions, which might sometimes come into conflict. In our example, Carol explains the requirements based on the contract, and on that basis justifies why Dave's lack of commitment to the plan may mean that he cannot continue in this service. Although the conflict seems unresolved, Carol does not "abandon" Dave by just guiding him out of the service to find other housing and support options. Instead, she suggests that a care planning meeting should be organised by the social worker who is responsible for the client's overall situation and the package of services. The participants at the meeting can include the client's family members and other professionals concerned, such as the client's psychiatrist from the health services and his social therapist from a substance abuse outpatient clinic. The core function of a meeting like this is to negotiate each stakeholder's responsibilities (or non-responsibilities) in finding new solutions, choices, resources and support arrangements in the client's current difficult situation.

The core concept of this book – responsibilisation – is present in several ways in Dave and Carol's conversation. Responsibilisation in its simplest sense means treating some individuals or groups of people (e.g. clients and workers) as having certain responsibilities and making efforts to get them to act according to these responsibilities. Responsibilisation of the client by the worker is the most obvious in the example: Carol makes it clear that the client should fulfil the obligations as stipulated in the care plan. Accordingly, as he has not acted as expected so far, he needs to start meeting the obligations he has agreed to. However, responsibilisation does not solely mean efforts to regulate others, but also oneself. In the example, Carol accomplishes self-responsibilisation in the sense that she justifies the demands on Dave in terms of her contract-based responsibilities towards the municipality. She explains to Dave that, according to the contract, clients should accept home visits and join group activities, and they should commit to abstinence from drugs and alcohol during the rehabilitation process. Whilst explaining this, she simultaneously displays herself as responsible for acting according to these expectations. Conversely, this self-responsibilisation is constructed as a consequence of responsibilisation targeted at the supported housing service by the purchaser. Dave, for his part, displays both self-responsibilisation and resistance towards expectations. He first gives an account of himself that suggests he has tried his best, and in that sense portrays himself as a responsible and "trying" person. After that, however, Dave excuses his apparent failures by placing blame on the lack of clarity in the care planning process and on too-high expectations in regard to his state of health. He also justifies his absence from certain service occasions by making apparent his discomfort with home visiting and group activities. In other words, he constructs the responsibilities set upon him as unsuitable and unreasonable in the current situation. Eventually, the example also implies responsibilisation targeted at absent parties: Carol suggests that the next step could be that Dave's social worker will organise a care planning meeting. There, the responsibilities of all the stakeholders for finding solutions and ways to proceed in the difficult situation can be negotiated and possibly reorganised.

Managing responsibilities between different parties is highly consequential for clients who are vulnerable and stigmatised, and suffer from complex problems. Who defines the responsibilities for supporting, helping and controlling the client, and on what grounds? What kinds of services are they assessed as being entitled to? What are their own positions and possibilities in negotiating responsibilities at various multi-party meetings? Furthermore, grass-roots level workers who are near to clients (such as the supported housing service worker in our example) are often regarded as being central to the negotiation of such last-resort service obligations: they can be delegated large responsibilities in regard to ensuring clients' lives and progress, but they are not necessarily given enough resources, possibilities and discretion to influence the contents of their work. This book concentrates on the management of responsibilities at the margins of welfare services, especially from the point of view of clients' and grass-roots level workers' responsibilisation and self-responsibilisation. In examining this, we treat workers and clients as active participants, who are able to negotiate their own and others' responsibilities and also to challenge and resist the practices of responsibilisation.

Responsibilisation at the margins of welfare services

The title locates the context of the book at the margins of welfare services. By this we refer to such services that are categorised as last-resort supporting, helping and controlling places in Western welfare states. In other words, they are not understood as universal in the sense that all citizens are expected to use them during the course of their life. These kinds of universal services include, for example, general health services, children's day care services or old people's services. Since services at the margins of welfare are culturally understood as being part of unusual or even deviant life courses, clienthood is often stigmatised. Furthermore, clients at the margins of welfare often have scarce resources and limited choices, and are therefore dependent on existing services and workers' support.

The marginal services can also be characterised as being targeted at socially excluded citizens with complex and multiple needs related, for example, to severe mental health and substance abuse problems, homelessness and criminality. Clients can have clienthoods in several services at the same time, and often move or are forced to move between them – a phenomenon known as "revolving door syndrome".

As the book's title suggests, by examining the margins of welfare services our focus is on responsibilisation. Above, we have defined it in an everyday sense, but in the social science literature it is a highly theorised concept. Its origin lies in Nikolas Rose and Peter Miller's writings on advanced liberalism and governmentality (e.g. Rose and Miller 1992; Rose 1999, 2000; Miller and Rose 2008), and the concept has been developed by a number of writers (e.g. Kemshall 2002; Clarke 2005; Bennett 2008; Ilcan 2009; O'Malley 2009; Brown and Baker 2012; Hansson *et al.* 2015; Peters 2016). According to this literature, clients are subjected to new kinds of responsibilisation as a result of welfare policy shifts in recent decades. Instead of the state taking the main responsibility for promoting citizens' well-being and providing services, increasingly this has become the primary responsibility of individuals, families and communities. It is not only clients but also welfare service providers and workers whose responsibilities have been under scrutiny. Their roles have changed considerably under the influence of managerialism, which is closely related to an advanced liberal way of governing. Welfare service providers and workers have become deeply responsibilised for the conduct, cost-effectiveness and outcomes of their work through a process called "new accountability" (e.g. Martin and Kettner 1997; Banks 2004; Saario 2014).

Building a bridge: responsibilisation in grass-roots level welfare practices

Whilst much has been written about the all-pervasive move to advanced liberal policies, the direct impact on workers and clients in terms of the actual, grass-roots level provision of welfare services is less clear. How do policies, procedures and organisational arrangements constrain and enable interaction between clients and welfare workers in the era of responsibilisation? Workers as grass-roots level practitioners mediate between state policies and clients' realities. They encounter clients face-to-face as a definitive part of their work and participate in institutional assessments and decision making about service provision and monitoring. They have been called "street level bureaucrats" (Lipsky 1980). Such workers have considerable power over the clients' lives, whilst at the same time they are themselves controlled by managers and institutional procedures. They are required to take on responsibility for professional practices that enable and produce independent and responsible citizenship. Clients, for their part, have responsibility to strengthen their independence and life management. This mutual "dependence" of welfare workers and clients makes it important to study the everyday negotiations and management of responsibilities from the point of view of both workers' and clients' responsibilisation and self-responsibilisation.

This book aims to build a bridge between more macro-level and theoretical literature concerning responsibilisation and grass-roots level practices at the margins of welfare services. This means studying the management of responsibilities by analysing in detail client–worker conversations, multi-party case-planning meetings, workers' team meetings and interviews with various stakeholders. In analysing these data, ethnomethodologically informed analytic concepts are applied that help to indicate subtle responsibilisation practices in welfare work. Mediating analytic concepts are needed, since the concept of responsibilisation as such is unlikely to appear in everyday language use by those whom it may concern. The data used in the book are mainly pertaining to Finnish and English supported housing and floating support services, targeted at people with complex mental health and substance abuse needs who are at risk of becoming homeless. As the clients of these services often use various other social and health services, the representatives of these other services, as well as municipal service purchasers, are also strongly present in the data.

There are several practical reasons why the data come mainly from England and Finland. Nevertheless, these two countries also form a reasonable pair in the sense that England has often been named as a forerunner in welfare state transformations, including a shift to an advanced liberal way of governing, whereas Finland can be described more as a follower although it has a strong history as a Nordic welfare state based on universalism. Despite this data concentration, we believe that this book's findings on responsibilisation in grass-roots level practices are largely recognisable at the margins of welfare services in other Western countries as well. This is because strong policy-level ideas on the changing roles of the state and citizens in welfare provision and promotion are applied and challenged currently across the Western world.

The organisation of the book

The book is organised so that the chapters form a coherent whole. Chapters 2–4 create theoretical, conceptual and methodological premises and reflective grounds for the subsequent empirically grounded chapters. Chapter 2 provides a short overview of governmentality literature from the point of view of the concept of responsibilisation. The review summarises the following interconnected themes by demonstrating the transformation of welfare states towards an advanced liberal way of governing:

- autonomy and choice
- enterprising selves
- governing at a distance.

It examines the managing of responsibilities as described in the literature from both citizens'/clients' and service providers'/welfare workers' perspectives, and how both parties are created as subjects of responsibility (the central viewpoint throughout the present book). Chapter 3 widens the discussion towards currently influential discourses on the new directions of Western welfare states by reviewing sociopolitical and professional literature concerning both welfare workers' and clients' expected roles in welfare services. It is demonstrated how responsibilities and responsibilisation are among the core topics not only in the governmentality literature, but also in the influential welfare discourses. Discourses are organised around such keywords as empowerment, participation, consumerism, personalisation, recovery and resilience. These welfare discourses both support and challenge the ideas presented in the governmentality literature. Chapter 4 constructs a methodological framework for the rest of the book, introducing first the premises of ethnomethodologically oriented research on grass-roots level practices. It then moves on to discuss how macro-level policies and policy transformations, and related welfare discourses, can be examined as human and interactional accomplishment in everyday welfare practices. After that, such analytic concepts are presented that are pertinent for analysing the management of responsibilities and responsibilisation. The analytic concepts introduced are responsibility, accountability, categorisation, boundary work, sequentiality, advice-giving, narrative and resistance. The chapter ends by briefly describing the welfare service settings and research material that are used in the subsequent chapters in studying welfare practices.

These chapters are followed by six analyses (Chapters 5–10) that approach responsibility management from a particular angle, by combining certain key ideas of responsibilisation and related welfare discourses, analytic concepts and research data. Together, these chapters create a comprehensive and multi-voiced picture of the responsibilisation practices at the margins of welfare services. These empirical chapters are briefly described below.

The first three of these chapters (5–7) concentrate on the management of clients' responsibilities. Chapter 5 demonstrates how on the one hand the interviewed clients at the margins of welfare services (try to) live up to the idea of the responsible self, and on the other hand resist this cultural expectation as impossible or unreasonable. It deepens self-responsibilisation discussions by first introducing the intertwined nature of a personal responsibility and social responsibility; and second by examining the dilemmatic nature of the currently strong self-management approach in mental health. It offers a contextually shifting and potentially empowering or discouraging framework for the client to make sense of the self in the middle of everyday struggles. Chapter 6 addresses the current topics – participation and "return to the community" – as interpreted in the discourse of active citizenship by examining client–worker interaction in mental health home visits and in prisons' pre-release meetings. It discusses how citizens are governed to become active and responsible members in the community, and shows what this means especially for those who confront the task of re-entering the community from institutional care and control settings. The analysis of the client–worker interaction demonstrates the joint activity of making active citizens at the grass-roots level welfare work. Chapter 7 focuses on life planning and case management by examining two case-planning meetings dealing with substance abuse, mental health and housing problems. It shows how workers and clients talk about clients' progress in their housing and lives and about becoming more aware and self-responsible in relation to available choices and anticipated risks. In both cases, progress is not going well and risks are high. However, the allocation of responsibility to address these risks is managed differently.

The next chapters (8–10) move on to study the management of workers' responsibilities. Chapter 8 concentrates on the ways welfare workers negotiate and reflect their everyday responsibilities in focus groups. Responsibilities are first discussed in the frame of the managerialisation of welfare services and professional ethics and then approached from the grass-roots level viewpoint through the concepts of ethics work and accountability. Analysis reveals that workers frequently describe how they use case-sensitive discretion, and how they give priority to clients' well-being and safety despite the managerial time limits and pressures to cut costs. When facing conflicting expectations, they define themselves first of all as responsible for responding to their clients' needs. Chapter 9 starts from the assumption that due to welfare workers' different back-grounds and a fragmented service structure, professional responsibilities are complex and under increasing negotiations. By analysing workers' collegial talk in team meetings, the chapter studies how they negotiate boundaries between their responsibilities and those of collaborative workers. It is found that bound-aries become increasingly negotiable when risks arise, for example when the cli-ent's mental well-being is worsening. In these situations, workers engage in boundary work by which they allocate responsibilities regarding who will act or who has the most relevant knowledge of the client. The focus of Chapter 10 is commissioning, which means a market-based arrangement where commissioners purchase services from the contracted providers. Drawing on interviews with commissioners, service provider managers and care coordinators, the chapter investigates service providers' responsibilities that relate to their contractual duties within commissioning. It is found that the commissioning system is based on a notion of progress, where the commissioners check that all parties remain on course to keep clients moving through the system. However, subtle resistance is voiced by service providers and care coordinators, especially towards this premise that is seen to hamper good quality everyday practices at the margins of welfare services.

References

Banks, S. (2004) *Ethics, Accountability and the Social Professions*, Basingstoke, UK: Palgrave Macmillan.

Bennett, J. (2008) "They hug hoodies, don't they? Responsibility, irresponsibility and responsibilisation in Conservative crime policy", *The Howard Journal of Criminal Justice*, 47(5): 451–469.

Brown, B.J. and Baker, S. (2012) *Responsible Citizens: Individuals, health and policy under neoliberalism*, London: Anthem Press.

Clarke, J. (2005) "New Labour's citizens: activated, empowered, responsibilized, aban-doned?", *Critical Social Policy*, 25(4): 447–463.

Hansson, S. and Hellberg, S. with Stern, M. (eds) (2015) *Studying the Agency of Being Governed*, London: Routledge.

Ilcan, S. (2009) "Privatizing responsibility: public sector reform under neoliberal government", *Canadian Review of Sociology*, 46(3): 207–234.

Kemshall, H. (2002) "Effective practice in probation: an example of 'advanced liberal' responsibilisation?", *The Howard Journal of Criminal Justice*, 41(1): 41–58.

Lipsky, M. (1980) *Street-level Bureaucracy: Dilemmas of the individual in public services*, New York: Russell Sage Foundation.

Martin, L.L. and Kettner, P.M. (1997) "Performance measurement: the new accountability", *Administration in Social Work*, 21(1): 17–29.

Miller, P. and Rose, N. (2008) *Governing the Present: Administering economic, social and personal life*, Cambridge: Polity Press.

O'Malley, P. (2009) "Responsibilization", in A. Wakefield and J. Fleming (eds) *The SAGE Dictionary of Policing* (pp. 277–279), London: Sage.

Peters, M.A. (2016) "From State responsibility for education and welfare to self-responsibilisation in the market", *Discourse: Studies in the Cultural Politics of Education*, DOI: 10.1080/01596306.2016.1163854.

Rose, N. (1999) *Powers of Freedom: Reframing political thought*, Cambridge: Cambridge University Press.

Rose, N. (2000) "Government and control", *The British Journal of Criminology*, 40(2): 321–339.

Rose, N. and Miller, P. (1992) "Political Power beyond the State: problematics of government", *British Journal of Sociology*, 43(2): 173–205.

Saario, S. (2014) *Audit Techniques in Mental Health: Practitioners' responses to electronic health records and service purchasing agreements*, Tampere: Acta Universitatis Tamperensis, 1907.

Part I

Conceptual and methodological premises

2 Responsibilisation in governmentality literature

Kirsi Juhila, Suvi Raitakari and Cecilia Hansen Löfstrand

Introduction

Responsibility is one of the concepts that has been intensively used and analysed in social sciences during the last three decades. In this chapter, our interest is primarily in responsibility literature that discusses responsibilities in regard to the changing roles of citizens, clients and providers in Western welfare societies. This interest brings us to the formulation of the concept that describes the claimed direction of this change, namely responsibilisation. Since the 1990s, this formulation has gradually become more and more common. As Brown and Baker (2012: 18) note, the concept of responsibilisation "is appearing with increasing frequency in accounts of management, social policy, health and welfare". The concept has also entered *The Sage Dictionary of Policing*, where O'Malley (2009: 277–279) defines it in the following way:

> "Responsibilization" is a term developed in the governmentality literature to refer to the process whereby subjects are rendered individually responsible for a task which previously would have been the duty of another – usually a state agency – or would not have been recognized as a responsibility at all. The process is strongly associated with neoliberal political discourses, where it takes on the implication that the subject being responsibilized has avoided this duty or the responsibility has been taken away from them in the welfare state era and managed by an expert or government agency.

This straightforward definition works as a good starting point for this book, which concentrates on the margins of welfare services. Our aim is, however, to bring more perspectives and nuances to responsibilisation by analysing the various ways it is accomplished and resisted in grass-roots level processes and practices. In this chapter we give a short overview of governmentality literature from the point of view of responsibilisation, which we use as a reflective ground for the forthcoming chapters. The chapter first deals with the origin of the responsibilisation concept and its main characteristics. It then proceeds, as described in the governmentality literature, to examine the concept from the perspectives of both citizens/welfare clients and service providers/workers.

Responsibilisation and advanced liberalism

Governmentality, advanced liberalism and neoliberalism

The governmentality literature concerning responsibilisation draws almost exclusively on the same origins. The roots of the concept are located in the writings of Rose and Miller (e.g. Rose 1990, 1999, 2000; Rose and Miller 1992; Miller and Rose 2008) and, through them, in Foucault's (e.g. 1977, 1982, 1988, 1991, 1997) notions on the new mode of governmentality, which is grounded in the conduct of conduct including the governance of others, self-governance and various technologies of self (see also Dean 1999; Lemke 2001; Rose *et al.* 2006; Cossman 2007, 2013; Houdt and Schinkel 2014). Lemke (2001: 191) makes a two-dimensional definition of governmentality based on Foucault's ideas:

> The term pin-points a specific form of *representation*; government defines a discursive field in which exercising power is "rationalized". This occurs, among other things, by the delineation of concepts, the specification of objects and borders, the provision of arguments and justifications, etc. In this manner, government enables a problem to be addressed and offers certain strategies for solving/handling the problem. On the other hand, it also structures specific forms of *intervention*. For a political rationality is not pure, neutral knowledge which simply "re-presents" the governing reality; instead, it itself constitutes the intellectual processing of the reality which political technologies can then tackle. This is understood to include agencies, procedures, institutions, legal forms, etc., that are intended to enable us to govern the objects and subjects of a political rationality. [Italics in original.]

Miller and Rose connect responsibilisation to a certain way of governing that they call "advanced liberalism". In response to the question, "What is it to govern in an advanced liberal way?" they answer (Miller and Rose 2008: 212) as follows:

> Over the closing decades of the twentieth century, "advanced liberal" strategies could be observed in national contexts from Finland to Australia, advocated by political regimes from left and right, and in relation to problem domains from crime control to health. They sought to develop techniques of government that created a distance between the decisions of formal political institutions and other social actors, conceived of these actors in new ways as subjects of responsibility, autonomy and choice, and hoped to act upon them through shaping and utilizing their freedom.

According to O'Malley (2009), the practices of responsibilisation are "strongly associated with neoliberal political discourses". Neoliberalism and advanced liberalism as described in the governmentality literature are thus connected to one another: neoliberalism, as a normative political rationality, is produced (in practice) according to an advanced liberal way of governing technologies, such as specific responsibility projects (Teghtsoonian 2009: 29). According to Cossman (2013: 895), "self-governance is a form of governance that has been particularly central in neoliberalism". However, neoliberalism is a political doctrine most often supported by conservative and right-wing parties, whilst the ideas of advanced liberalism have spread across different Western democratic countries and have been promoted by parties from the left and right (Miller and Rose 2008: 212). For this reason, to comprehensively cover the various dimensions of the responsibilisation discourses, we prefer using the concept of advanced liberalism instead of neoliberalism, although the latter concept is also widely used in the governmentality literature.

Autonomy and choice

Advanced liberalism is based on "a new specification of the subject of government": that is, on the expectation of individuals to be active in their own government instead of passive and dependent, and to conduct their lives like enterprises (Rose and Miller 1992: 198–199; Rose 1999: 164–165). Accordingly, novel political and legal practices and techniques have emerged and developed that seek to support the cultivation and development of self-governing "actively responsible subjects" (Barnett 2003). Responsibility is closely connected to autonomy and choice. Citizens in advanced liberal societies are supposed to (and are also directed to) make such choices that maximise their well-being, health, safety and quality of life. It is through making individual choices in their personal everyday lives, and in their various encounters with other people in workplaces, neighbourhoods, social and health services and so on, that individuals are seen to fulfil their national obligations. However, the problem is whether this expanding freedom of choice is used responsibly and, if not, how (i.e. by what means) to govern individuals towards more responsible choices (Miller and Rose 2008: 204, 213–214). As such, the aim of advanced liberalism is to create governance techniques that are directed to the "management of freedom" and to "link subjects to their own subjection" (Barnett 2003: 31; Brown 2012).

Subject responsibilisation in an advanced liberal way of governing is inherently dilemmatic and paradoxical, including both empowering and manipulating elements (Hodgson 2001; van der Land 2014: 426). On the one hand, individuals are supposed to voluntarily conduct their own lives responsibly. But on the other hand, they "will have to make their decisions about their self-conduct surrounded by a web of vocabularies, injunctions, promises, dire warnings and threats of intervention, organized increasingly around a proliferation of norms and normativities" (Miller and Rose 2008: 205). Responsibilisation is thus not the same as total freedom of choice, but there are certain rules and boundaries based, for instance, on legislation or on expert knowledge on a good and healthy life and way of being (Brown and Baker 2012: 19). Citizens who are assessed to have broken the rules and boundaries of active citizenship by making unreasonable or unmoral choices in their lives make the dilemma related to responsibilisation clearly visible. As Tonkens (2011: 61) argues, responsibilisation and de-responsibilisation co-occur. The "irresponsible" citizens' autonomy and free choice are often restricted, and they become subjugated to various re-responsiblisation techniques and procedures that include, among other things, sanctions accompanied by schemes for "naming, shaming and blaming" (Rose 2000: 322).

Enterprising selves

Self-entrepreneurship means that individuals are expected to invest in themselves to develop their social abilities and to work on their well-being and health. All these developments are distinctive of the discourse of individual responsibilisation (Teghtsoonian 2009: 29; Broom *et al.* 2014: 516). Rational choice-making concerning one's life is the core of the responsibilisation discourse. Clarke (2005: 451), in his analysis on British New Labour's policies concerning citizenship, writes about "the responsibilized citizens" who must exercise their autonomy and freedom responsibly by making reasonable and right choices. Clarke (2005: 451) continues to state that this demand includes a moralistic point, since "unreasonable" choices are interpreted rather as the acts of an irresponsible citizen than as the consequences of structural inequalities and a lack of opportunities. This kind of moral emphasis is characteristic of advanced liberal governmentality in general and of its techniques of responsibilisation that are fundamentally based on entrepreneurial moral agency (Shamir 2008: 7).

An economic logic constitutes the base of the advanced liberal way of governing. As Rose (1999: 141–142) writes, "all aspects of *social* behaviour are now reconceptualised along economic lines – as calculative actions undertaken through the universal human faculty of choice" (italics in original), and "all manner of social undertakings – health, welfare, education, insurance – can be reconstructed in terms of their contribution to the development of human capital" (see also Lemke 2001: 197, 202–203). According to this logic, individuals are defined as rational calculative actors or as "enterprising selves", who, by comparing costs and benefits, make the best possible choices from the point of view of themselves and their families.

Governing at a distance

One of the core consequences of the responsibilisation in advanced liberalism is claimed to be that it reorganises state–citizens and state–local responsibilities in a way that is described as governing at a distance (Dean 1999; Lemke 2001; Barnett 2003; Miller and Rose 2008). In social and health care services, this has meant a shift from a provision-based paradigm to a framework-based paradigm. In other words, instead of both steering and rowing, the state merely steers (Carney 2008: 102). This highlights the transition in public service delivery in two senses. First (as described above), instead of the state taking the main responsibility for social and health policies by promoting the well-being of citizens and tackling inequalities and exclusion, these have become the primary responsibilities of individuals, families and communities (Bennett 2008: 454–455; Lister 2015). Second, not only the responsibilities of citizens as clients but also the responsibilities of local-level service providers and non-governmental organisations (NGOs) have been renegotiated (Osbourne and Gaebler 1993; Healy 2009; Ilcan 2009). Hence, governing in an advanced liberal way entails new constellations of partnerships between public, private and voluntary actors (Thörn and Larsson 2012: 264–266).

Responsibilities are allocated increasingly to the local, civil society level that Ilcan and Basok (2004: 130) call "community government" (see also Lister 2015: 363–364). As Goddard (2012: 351) describes, this tendency is taking place in, for example, crime prevention:

> The thinking was that the Government cannot – or should not – be solely responsible for reducing crime rates. Rather, community safety and crime prevention has been devolved from a centralized authority to local community partnerships, and carried out by local community-based organizations.

Governing at a distance also means that local service providers and professionals are increasingly commissioned and monitored (and thus responsibilised) for the content and outcomes of services (Ilcan and Basok 2004; Dent 2006). In addition, the state's role as a provider of services has decreased and its roles as an allocator of resources and as a manager of contracts have increased, as service provision has been handed more to the commercial and third-sector actors (Bennett 2008: 465). For instance, as a result of major changes in housing policy in Sweden during the 1990s (Sahlin 2004), the responsibility for providing housing for the homeless was transferred from the state and municipal housing companies to the local social authorities. The state has thus "rolled back", but it has not ceased to govern or "steer". As shown by Sahlin (2004: 346–348, 362–363), the means for governing have been altered. The Swedish state now governs at a distance through discourse and project funding. It governs through discourse when defining and attaching meaning to homelessness as a term and phenomenon (by, for example, compiling, producing and disseminating knowledge about it). It governs through project funding when stipulating the target groups of the projects entitled to apply for and to be taken into consideration as possible recipients of funding.

Citizens and welfare clients as subjects of responsibility

Active citizenship and the privatisation of risks

The advanced liberal way of governing goes hand in hand with changes that emphasise active citizenship instead of dependency on welfare states. Newman and Tonkens (2011: 9) conclude that active citizenship has three related dimensions:

- the possibility of making choices about one's welfare services;
- individuals', families' and communities' increasing responsibility for welfare;
- participation in collaborative governance, such as community-based policy-making and service planning.

What unifies these dimensions is the idea that individual citizens and local communities should take a greater role in society in regard to the creation of well-being, health and safety, and should not expect welfare to be created or social problems to be solved top-to-bottom by the welfare state. This premise resonates well with the idea of a "Big Society," which is based originally on British new conservatism that favours a strong civil society and private companies instead of a strong, interventionist state or government (Pathak 2013: 62; MacKinnon and Derickson 2013: 262–263; Lister 2015). As Lister (2015: 361) states, "A central theme of the Big Society agenda is an emphasis upon responsibility. Yet this emphasis is far from new".

Miller and Rose (2008: 214–215) approach the above described changes in welfare states as a shift from a social insurance principle ("socialised forms of risk management") to a privatisation of risk management. By this they mean that citizens can no longer trust and rely on the welfare state providing them with help and resources when they face unemployment, fall ill, become old and so on. Instead, insurance against these kinds of future risks and prospects becomes defined as the private concerns and responsibilities of citizens. Lemke (2001: 201) follows the same line of interpretation by arguing that social risks (such as illness, unemployment and poverty) have been transformed into problems of "self-care" (see also Cossman 2013: 896). Citizen responsibilisation is thus linked to the retreat and "irresponsibilisation" of state and public government (Cradock 2007: 162; Liebenberg *et al.* 2015: 1007). This kind of increasing ignorance of the structural roots of problems and the privatisation of the risks of unemployment and other significant areas in people's everyday lives (such as housing) are studied and recognised widely in Western countries (e.g. Whiteford 2010; Solberg 2011; Lantz and Marston 2012; Stonehouse *et al.* 2015). For example, Lantz and Marston (2012) study the shift from socialised to private risk management in an Australian context. They do so from the point of view of how disabled persons previously seen as deserving of government support are now included in the expanding category of "undeserving citizens" whose worth is validated primarily through active and self-responsible labour market participation. Instead of aiming to increase the number of available jobs, the idea is to promote such responsible citizenship, which includes "job readiness" and the obligation to work.

The privatisation of risk management means that citizens are expected to calculate their futures in the light of their present life choices and the risks related to them – such as what smoking or certain eating habits do to their health, what consequences interrupting vocational schooling might have, or how big a bank loan they dare to take if establishing a business of their own. An important skill in active citizenship is thus an ability to notice, calculate and reflect on future risks and to make reasonable life choices based on this ability. So, "responsibility for risks is increasingly devolved to individuals: risks are something that should be taken (an entrepreneurial attitude towards life is rewarded), but also prudently reflected upon" (Roberts 2006: 56). Thörn and Larsson (2012: 265–266) summarise this transformation as follows:

> This fundamental responsibility of the subject, emerging from the steering rationalities and practices of liberal engineering, also implies that the individual to a much higher degree than under the era of social engineering is considered responsible for putting her/himself in a situation in which s/he is in need of certain welfare transfers (related to unemployment, sickness and so on), since it is seen as *a consequence of past (bad) choices*. [Italics in original.]

Self-governing citizens and communities

The governmentality literature emphasises that in order to be able to reflect on risks and to make reasonable life choices – to become self-governing citizens – individuals are supposed to seek and use actively available expert knowledge and various educative material related to a rational, good and healthy way of living (Cossman 2013: 896). This responsibility to reflect on risks and to make reasonable choices has created demand for various forms of public and private counselling, such as governmental instructions for good eating and the appropriate level of physical exercise, educative television shows on people who follow expert advice on some aspects of their lives to reach better self-management, guidebooks and other self-help manuals for different areas of life, private therapists and trainers. Educational material and expert knowledge supporting self-management and self-surveillance are also increasingly being delivered for the clients in public health and social services. For example, in a study of the work of staff at a rehabilitative unit of the Swedish Public Employment Service, Garsten and Jacobsson (2013: 826) argue that the (normal) job-seeking citizen is "expected to actively assume responsibility for her own employability by being prepared to work on herself in order to improve her attractiveness to the labour market". Furthermore, they ask what happens to individuals who do not live up to this expectation and are then referred to job centres and rehabilitative units.

In creating self-governing citizens, the main question and message are as follows: "What can you do to help yourself?" and "You have to do it yourself and make plans for your future." Juhila *et al.* (2015) discuss how clients are supported and directed to become self-governing citizens in the community mental health practitioner–client interactions in a Finnish supported housing unit, by encouraging them to make weekly schedules of their activities and to regularly attend activities in the community (i.e. to integrate themselves into the community). Community mental health work can thus be interpreted as an endeavour to work on the self with the intention of creating more active citizens (see also Raitakari *et al.* 2015). This kind of problem solving by strengthening the abilities of people to govern their conduct, minds and destinies has particularly created markets for such "psy-professions" that are seen to have the therapeutic expertise to help individuals to work on themselves (Rose 1999: 89–93; Cossman 2013: 896).

Counselling and education seeking to reinforce self-governmentality have a future orientation and causal logic, in the sense that citizens are reminded that various life choices "here and now" will have consequences for individuals' well-being in the forthcoming years and through whole lifespans. So, learning to make the right, knowledge-based choices now reduces certain risks, prevents problems and ensures a better quality of life in the future (Juhila *et al.* 2015). Making non-risky choices concerning personal health, and via that preventing otherwise threatening illnesses, is the most obvious area of life where this time-related and causal self-responsibilisation idea is present in current policies and discussions in Western welfare societies (e.g. Michailakis and Schirmer 2010; Brown 2013). As Peeters (2013: 588) writes about the Dutch government health policy discourse: "on the one hand, the responsibility of citizens for their own health is left untouched … on the other hand, government presumes a healthy lifestyle to be a rational choice and the social norm". All in all, citizens are expected to plan and ensure their whole lifespans responsibly: for instance, to prepare for good ageing and old age by making the right housing and financial choices and by creating good social safety networks early enough (cf. active and positive ageing) (Asquith 2009; Anttonen and Häikiö 2011), and furthermore to not conduct criminal acts or use substances abusively since they may cause serious troubles in citizens' future lives. This leads to a belief that illness and social problems are caused by "bad behaviour", and that citizens need to be advised (moralised) and educated to choose (by their own free will) a better (more responsible) way of living and behaving (Brown 2012, 2013).

In advanced liberalism, responsibility for self-government is claimed to include not only personal self-management; self-governed citizens are also made responsible for the welfare of family members and community members, and even for participating in sustainable policymaking at a wider societal level (Houdt and Schinkel 2014; Lister 2015). Cossman (2013: 898) writes about the changing role of families as follows: "responsibilization within the family has taken on a new intensity, with a renewed demand on families to meet the needs of its members from child care to health care to welfare" (see also Cossman 2007: 11; Treloar and Funk 2008; Dahlstedt and Fejes 2014; Trnka 2014). At a community level, the slogan "everybody has a responsibility" invites neighbours, volunteers and NGOs "to work in roles once performed by states, or in some development contexts, in the ongoing absence of state-supported social service institutions" (Lacey and Ilcan 2006: 47). This community responsibilisation (Silverstein and Spark 2007: 339) also comprises expectations to deal with difficult health and social issues – such as mental health problems, criminality, homelessness and violence – at the local level, that is to say, among "ordinary" community members (Hörnqvist 2001; May *et al.* 2005: 717; Muncie 2006: 773; Silverstein and Spark 2007; van der Land 2014; Lister 2015).

"Irresponsible" citizens and responsibility projects

Expectations to become self-governing citizens concern all citizens and communities in advanced liberalism. However, special attention is targeted at individuals and groups who are assessed as having special difficulties in managing risks and becoming self-responsible. So, for citizens defined as having difficulties in becoming enterprising selves, there is a growing tendency to develop various institutional and professional enabling programmes that seek to strengthen individuals' responsibilities for their own lives (e.g. Jayasuriya 2002). The programmes are foremost targeted at vulnerable, disadvantaged and socially excluded people who live and have clienthoods at the margins of welfare services, such as mental health, substance abuse, probation and homelessness services.

Ilcan (2009: 220–221) calls the aforementioned programmes that target people at the margins of welfare services "responsibility projects". He connects them to the idea of governing at a distance in the sense that the projects are "practiced, exercised, and carried out through numerous governments, organizations, and programs that aim to make certain groups more responsible for transforming their conduct", rather than passing down authoritative regulations and orders from a "big" state. As the emphasis is on individual conduct, training and education, the projects move the focus away from structural exclusion and explanations. In other words, the focus is on the lifestyle changes of welfare clients instead of on tackling societal and economic inequalities (Ferguson 2007: 395–397; Scoular and O'Neill 2007: 770–771). This resonates with the claim that respective societies should not encourage welfare dependency but meet it with zero tolerance (Ramon 2008: 117; Cossman 2007: 12; Pollack 2010: 1266). However, focusing on individuals and treating them as autonomous actors is in contrast with the idea (largely shared, for instance, among social and health care researchers and front-level workers) that social ecological contexts and their processing are significant when aiming to improve the living situations of the most vulnerable citizens and their possibility of making choices (e.g. Brown 2013; Liebenberg *et al.* 2015: 1007).

Responsibility projects are a reality for people involved with the criminal justice system or for people making claims for assistance from the state – for example, those applying for social assistance, unemployment or medical benefits (Pollack 2010). Pollack (2010: 1271–1272) discusses the governing of marginality and "risky clients" based on an interview study concerning women in Canada who had former experiences of incarceration. She expresses reservations in terms of how the women – who are disempowered through poverty, violence and racialisation – are managed by institutions and professionals, as if the cause of their problems is an inability to govern their own lives. The interviewed women pointed out that the perspectives of welfare professionals (despite emphasising individual empowerment as a pronounced aim) left little or no room for their own subjective views. Emotional, attitudinal and psychological factors were evaluated as part of the risk assessment, and individual responsibility was valorised, whereas "important factors such as poverty, violence against women, lack of community support, stigmatization and barriers to unemployment" were ignored (Pollack 2010: 1271–1272).

Individual responsibility projects construct welfare clients' past lives as unsuccessful, or as a series of failures, based on bad or irresponsible choices that have caused the unfortunate and troubling present situation. In other words, they have taken risks that they have not been able to govern themselves, and "irresponsibility" might also have caused problems and danger for other citizens and for the whole of society. Projects aim both to make individuals see and admit personal failures and to create their capacity to avoid failures and to make better choices in the future. Since the focus is on personal failures, bad choices and unnecessary risks taken, the projects have a strong moral dimension (Kemshall 2002: 44; Muncie 2006: 780–781). Rose (2000: 334) writes:

> Within these new politics of conduct, the problems of problematic persons are reformulated as moral or ethical problems, that is to say, problems in the ways in which such persons understand and conduct themselves and their existence. This ethical reformulation opens the possibility for a whole range of psychological techniques to be recycled in programmes for governing "the excluded". The imperative of activity, and the presupposition of an ethic of choice, is central not only to rationale of policy but also to the reformatory technology to which it is linked.

Ethical reformulation in the sense of learning to make better life choices and to avoid personal failures in the future includes the message that we all have to stop blaming others, the government or society for our own misfortune, problems and failures (Silverstein and Spark 2007: 332; Kemshall 2008: 21–22). Instead we have to recognise and confront that our own ways of thinking, our acts and our behaviour are the cause of the troubles. For instance, Lyon-Callo's (2000: 328) ethnographic study of an emergency shelter in Massachusetts illustrates how the dominant discursive practices based on diagnosing and treating the individual selves aim to produce "homeless subjects who learn to look within their selves for the cause of their homelessness".

Not blaming others, accepting our responsibility and working on ourselves are all seen as ways to achieve personal autonomy and freedom and to become self-governing, rational and moral choice-makers (Rose 2000: 334). This empowering of the self has another side of the coin that can be called a "blaming the victim" strategy (Gray 2009: 330), which bypasses structural inequalities and individuals' vulnerabilities connected to, for instance, violence and mental health problems. This critique is highly relevant when taking into account that responsibility measures, projects and programmes are carried out especially among marginalised citizens – such as battered women, people with mental health problems, illegal drug users, homeless people or (young) offenders – who often have the most disadvantaged position in society and restricted possibilities of choice-making (May *et al.* 2005; Silverstein and Spark 2007; Ramon 2008; Fischer and Neale 2008; Whiteford 2010; Barry 2013).

Responsibility projects also produce divisions into "not to be blamed" and "blamed", "deserved" and "undeserved" client categories (e.g. Barnett 2003; Lantz and Marston 2012). For instance, Hansen Löfstrand (2012b) argues that homelessness services share a tendency to draw boundaries between "the truly homeless" and the rest. The latter should be or should have been able to take responsibility for their housing situation and become responsible. In contrast, "the truly homeless" are categorised as suffering from an "incurable illness" due to severe social or medical problems. Since they are not expected to be able to become self-responsible, they are not blamed for their homelessness and are seen as eligible for permanent homeless accommodation. This narrowing of the category of "the (truly) homeless" rests on a medicalisation of homelessness. It also bypasses structural explanations and increases the self-responsibilisation expectations and blaming of the homeless, who are defined as capable of improving their life situation.

Accepting responsibility for one's past choices and failures is logically followed by taking responsibility for future life choices and paths. The core aim of the projects at the margins of welfare is thus to make clients understand that they themselves are ultimately responsible for their improvement (Lynch 2000: 40). Clients are supported and given tools for reaching this aim during the projects, but in the future they should manage on their own. And if they fail again, the project is not to be blamed first but rather the clients themselves. Silverstein and Spark (2007: 338) and Liebenberg *et al.* (2015: 1007) comment on the unfairness of this – the credit for success goes easily to the projects but the blame for failure goes to the clients, because the responsibility for failure is not likely to be attributed to the projects and their practices.

Rose (2000: 335) claims that in advanced liberalism "those who refuse to become responsible, to govern themselves ethically, have also refused the offer to become members of our moral community. Hence, for them, harsh measures are entirely appropriate." Different responsibility projects are such "harsh measures", but even harsher measures can be targeted at those who, despite getting the opportunity to participate in such projects, do not learn self-government and fail repeatedly (Barnett 2003: 30). As Tony Blair stated in 1997, whilst the Prime Minister of the United Kingdom: "Don't be surprised if the penalties are tougher when you have been given the opportunities but don't take them" (Muncie 2006: 782). In the end, the citizenship rights of those who have not taken opportunities might become conditional (Rose 2000: 335; Kemshall 2008: 31), meaning exclusion from some welfare services or even the partial denial of health treatment. These excluded are no longer highly prioritised cases (cf. Michailakis and Schirmer 2010) but can, in certain cases, even be called abandoned citizens (Clarke 2005). Butler and Benoit (2015: 28) argue that the

attainment of citizenship is fragile as it can be taken away if and when marginalised individuals do not act like good citizens. The moral component of citizenship is evident as it is up to the individual whether or not he or she will be seen by others (especially those in positions of power) as a citizen.

Responsibility projects can be successful in strengthening welfare clients' self-government, autonomy and ability to make better-informed life choices in the future. However, the more emphasis is placed on failures, bad choices and (self-)blaming excluded citizens, the more those getting blamed or blaming themselves have to carry societal stigmas. Consequently, "the demarcation of those who can play a full role in the welfare society from those who cannot" increases (Kemshall 2002: 41; see also Houdt and Schinkel 2014: 59–60).

Responsibilisation is not only a project to educate and modify citizens and welfare clients, but it is also to match the identities of workers and service providers to advanced liberal ideas of governance. We turn next to this other angle of responsibilisation.

Welfare workers and providers as subjects of responsibility

Managerialisation and new accountability

The role of social and health care professionals has changed considerably under the influence of New Public Management (NPM). This change is based on the ideas of advanced liberalism, closely related to managerialist market ideologies (Rose 1999: 151–153). Numerato *et al.* (2012: 629) conclude that "in the context of governmentality managerialisation represents a new mentality of the 'conduct of conduct' and provides a new invisible and all-pervasive technology to govern professionals". Kolthoff *et al.* (2007) identify two principles of NPM: managers gain control over professional practice, but this occurs in indirect ways rather than through direct authority (cf. governing at a distance). These indirect ways include:

- emphasising entrepreneurship and downsizing (e.g. privatisation, outsourcing and market models);
- decentralisation (e.g. local budgets and individually-tailored and costed services) performance management (e.g. auditing, contracts, targets and timetables);
- planning and control cycles (e.g. feedback systems, assessment and review systems, and information and communications technologies).

In other words, professionals have been deeply responsibilised for the conduct, cost-effectiveness and outcomes of their work (e.g. Power 1997; Dent 2006). This is called "new accountability" (Banks 2004; Martin and Kettner 1997; Saario 2014).

Le Bianic (2011: 803) concludes that the shift towards managerialism has eroded the traditional "foundation of professionalism based on client trust, autonomy of practice and collegial discipline". Professional responsibility has been replaced by professionals' accountability for the outcomes of their work based on organisational and contractual demands and expectations (Saario and Stepney 2009; Le Bianic 2011). Like entrepreneurs in businesses, professionals are held personally responsible and accountable for their work and possible failures in it, such as not successfully following the limits or budgets or not doing enough productive and effective preventive or rehabilitation work. They are also expected to personally and willingly align business principles in order to create self-responsible entrepreneurial identities (Keddie 2015). This kind of managerialist responsibilisation of grass-roots level workers has spread to all human service work, including work at the margins of welfare services.

The split between governmental/municipal service purchasers and service providers is an essential element in managerialism and strengthens market ideologies. The split means that one party commits to buying services under certain conditions, whilst the other party commits to producing them. The co-operation between the parties is grounded in contracts that explicate service providers' obligations to produce specified services for a certain group and number of citizens. Contracts might also contain bonuses for the successful production of services and sanctions for not fulfilling the obligations. The split into purchasers and providers can be internal in the sense that providers are governmental/municipal organisations and workers, who make contracts with governmental/municipal service purchasing organisations. Another option is an external purchaser–provider model that usually includes a tendering process organised by local governments as an aim to get service contracts with the best value. Both internal and external models follow the same logic of market-based governance and new accountability.

Service providers in the external purchaser–provider model can be private companies and NGOs. NGOs have long histories in welfare services in Western welfare states. They often target services to the most vulnerable and marginalised citizens, such as disabled people, people with mental health and substance abuse problems and homeless people. During recent decades, market-based governance, especially funding based on tendering and contracts, has changed their role significantly. For instance, in Sweden and Finland the introduction of a new system of pricing in many municipalities, starting in the 1990s, brought a new responsibilisation of NGOs as the providers of homelessness services. The new pricing system, based on the purchaser–provider model, means that the municipal administration purchases a product – temporary accommodation and support – regardless of whether the provider is municipal, a non-profit NGO or a for-profit provider (Bergmark 2001; Trydegård 2001; Hansen Löfstrand 2012a). The NGOs, like any other providers, are then paid per "full bed". Before the system of transfer pricing was introduced, they received a lump sum of money for running their services without continuous controls as to whether or to what extent their services were used. NGOs are increasingly challenged to demonstrate accountability, reporting the relevance and effectiveness of the produced services, as purchasers monitor and evaluate that the NGOs fulfil their contractual obligations (May *et al.* 2005: 715; Buckingham 2009: 235; Saario and Raitakari 2010; Hansen Löfstrand 2012a; Mueller-Hirth 2012; Juhila and Günther 2013).

Risk management and prevention

Besides the increased "new accountability", the advanced liberal way of governing has been argued to have produced other consequences for the roles of social and health care workers and service providers and the content of their work. One such change is that managing and preventing risks is emphasised as a significant responsibility of grass-roots level workers (Pollack 2010; Goddard 2012). Workers occupy the space between the state on the one hand, and individuals, families and communities on the other (Pollack 2010: 1263). They are responsible for identifying, assessing and managing "risky" individuals and families departing from "risk thinking" and cultivating a "risk gaze" (Rose 2000: 331–334). This new responsibility is bound to the ideas of the risk society (Beck 1992, 1999). The risk society demands that citizens take a calculative stance on their future opportunities and risks in the world of uncertainties and, on the basis of calculation, make the best possible life choices. This same logic is applicable to welfare workers and service providers in regard to their work. They are expected to adopt "risk thinking" and make the right assessments when identifying certain individuals or groups of citizens as "risky clients". On the basis of risk assessments, they should make justified decisions about whether and what kind of services to deliver, and about what support and control interventions to put into practice in order to prevent the worsening of the clients' situations and to prevent risks from being actualised (Pollack 2010).

Preventing risks means that the focus of work is on the present signs of concern, aiming to avoid future threats, problems, disasters and costs both at individual and societal levels (Parton 2006; Satka *et al.* 2011; Goddard 2012). Early intervention is the concept that is often in use when presenting this kind of risk-preventing work. Early intervention projects and related professional practices have been created especially to pinpoint children at risk (of different forms of abuse and/or deviant behaviour, and of exclusion in later life) at an early enough stage. To be successful, this kind of early intervention work is argued to need co-operation between different agencies such as schools, the police, maternity clinics, health centres and the social services concerning, for instance, information exchange on depicted concerns and planning measures to decrease risks. Not only do various professionals and welfare workers have a responsibility to observe and act on signs of concern, but all citizens – for example, people at workplaces and in neighbourhoods – are expected to participate, at least in so far as locating and intervening in urgent risks that need common attention. Thus, according to advanced liberalism, we all have a responsibility to ensure safer and healthier communities.

Although we all have a responsibility in preventing and managing risks, some groups of professionals and welfare workers carry a more central role in this – such as child protection, mental health and probation workers. These responsibilities relate especially to the individual cases that they have been working with. They are expected to assess the risks of such serious incidents as violence towards children, suicidal acts and so on occurring. This responsibility for anticipating tragic events and disasters becomes clearly visible if these kinds of incidents happen. The reasons for the disasters are then easily located in the failures of individual professionals (for not noticing and assessing the risks in the right way and in time). In public discussion, this kind of failure and blaming talk is often used when tragic events such as a school massacre are reported and dealt with. Accordingly, it is often argued that a tragic, incomprehensible event was conducted by a "risky" and "sick" person, who (according to criticism) had not been identified early enough or assessed and treated correctly by mental health or other involved professionals. Yet, welfare workers' responsibility for conducting risk assessment work is not only linked to serious threats; it is involved in their everyday work concerning "smaller scale risks", such as assessing whether the client in question is able to control their drinking, or to take care of their personal money matters next week or in the longer run and, if not, what kinds of interventions are needed.

All in all, the work of managing and preventing risk includes locating, supporting, directing, helping and controlling citizens at risk, and has wider aims to protect all citizens against the problems and threats that might be caused by "risky populations". In criminal policies this is called "new penology" (Feeley and Simon 1992). By referring to Feeley and Simon (1992), Le Bianic (2011: 807; see also Muncie 2006: 776) writes that, in this new approach, the task has changed from transformative to managerial: "This approach is no longer concerned with reducing crime through social programmes or rehabilitative efforts, but is mainly aimed at 'managing' criminal populations, protecting society and preventing risks of re-offending." This kind of risk management and prevention logic is widely in use at the margins of welfare services.

Re-educating and producing responsible citizens

Besides identifying risks, assessing them and making correctly timed interventions in high-risk situations and cases, welfare service providers and workers are expected to contribute to the creation of self-governing and responsible citizens in general. Experts and professionals fulfil this responsibility by presenting good life instructions and advice in various public forums (on television news and talk shows, in newspapers and magazines, on internet sites and social media etc.). There are a variety of authorised sources of knowledge and expertise on what advice and instructions for good citizenship and life-management are based on: from governmental sources (for example, representatives of ministries) and research knowledge (for example, representatives of health sciences), via professionals (doctors, psychologists, therapists, social workers etc.) to numerous experts-by-experience (people with self-made successful lives, recovered alcoholics or previously overweight people etc.). The responsibility of these holders of good life expertise is to convince citizens that they can and ought to choose a healthier and happier life by persistently following the given instructions and advice.

In addition to this general and public responsibilisation of citizens, self-governing individuals are expected to be educated via more personalised contacts in such governmental/municipal special institutions as schools, health centres and maternal clinics. Share and Strain (2008: 236) write about the "responsibilization of schools". By this they mean the increasing duties of school staff to personally "educate" not only children but also their parents. For example, the staff are expected to advise parents on the right food and nutrition for their children that supports the overall goal of producing responsible parenthood. This kind of educative work is well in line with the aim of the early intervention strategy described above.

The third and most direct level of being responsible for producing responsible citizens includes work in those institutions that deal with people who are assessed to have taken irresponsible risks and made wrong or bad choices (cf. responsibility projects). This kind of work is often done with long-term unemployed people, (former) prisoners, people with mental health and substance abuse problems and homeless people – in other words, people at the margins of welfare services. Clients at the margins of welfare settings are regarded as being in need of re-education. Hence, welfare workers' responsibilities include undertaking clients' re-education with the aim of enabling and producing independent and active citizenship. The clients, for their part, have a responsibility to strengthen their independence and capacities in order to be able to make better risk assessments and life choices in the future. In this sense, the workers and clients are mutually dependent, since the clients have to help the workers to help themselves (Matarese 2009). Clients who do not participate in this helping of workers might be in danger of being excluded from services due to being defined as unmotivated clients.

Institutions with specific client (re-)responsibilisation obligations are as accountable for the outcomes and cost-effectiveness of their work as any other social and health care services. To fulfil these obligations, structured and focused rehabilitation and training programmes have been developed, such as cognitive-behavioural programmes used, for example, in prisons, whose effectiveness has been demonstrated in evidence-based research on what works and what does not work (Muncie 2006: 776–777; Teghtsoonian 2009: 32).

Conclusion and discussion

In this chapter we have reviewed the governmentality literature from the point of view of how it deals with the concept of responsibilisation in the context of the advanced liberal way of governing. Our special focus has been on the developments and consequences of the concept at the margins of welfare services. As we have demonstrated, responsibilisation is an umbrella concept that includes a variety of meanings, interpretations and characteristics concerning the state, communities, citizens, welfare clients and workers, service providers and purchasers, and their relationships. The concept has been developed and applied in examining the preferred ways of being active, accountable and good actors in advanced liberalism.

The literature dealing with advanced liberalism and especially responsibilisation takes a critical stance. It leads to exploring the relationship between governance techniques, power relations, subjectivity and agency (Rasmussen 2011). Responsibilisation discourse is characterised as normative by its nature, and especially as a political programme it can be understood foremost as a moral project targeted at constituting self-governing subjects. Responsibilisation is defined in a critical light, especially from the point of view of the margins of welfare. It is claimed to produce, for instance, victim blaming and even the abandonment of "irresponsible" citizens. It is also often described as the prevailing and undesirable trend in Western welfare societies and in the globalising world in general.

The governmentality literature attributes the following core characteristics to the responsibilisation discourse:

- autonomy and choice
- enterprising selves
- governing at a distance.

These characteristics match and are relevant for both citizens/welfare clients and welfare workers/providers as the subjects of responsibility. We summarised the following emphases of citizens' and welfare clients' responsibilisation:

- active citizenship and the privatisation of risks
- self-governing citizens and communities
- "irresponsible" citizens and responsibility projects.

Welfare workers' and service providers' responsibilisation, on the other hand, is discussed in the literature from the following angles:

- managerialisation and new accountability
- risk management and prevention
- re-educating and producing responsible citizens.

Although the governmentality literature can be regarded as rather theoretical and abstract, it also provides an analytical toolbox for empirical research. As Rose *et al.* (2006: 101) write:

> we need to investigate the role of the grey sciences, the minor professions, the accountants and insurers, the managers and psychologists, in the mundane business of governing everyday economic and social life, in the shaping of governable domains and governable persons, in the new forms of power, authority and subjectivity being formed within these mundane practices.

Accordingly, this book aims to examine whether and how responsibilisation is present in the everyday realities and struggles of citizens, welfare clients and workers by analysing in detail texts, talk and interactions at the margins of welfare services. In doing this we add an ethnomethodologically oriented approach to the gradually growing empirical research on governmentality and responsibilisation (e.g. Colvin *et al.* 2010; Pollack 2010; Whiteford 2010; Rasmussen 2011; Solberg 2011; Brown 2012; Goddard 2012; Lantz and Marston 2012; Broom *et al.* 2014; Gradin Franzén 2015; Juhila *et al.* 2015; Berger 2015; Berger and Eskelinen 2016). In the end, it is the communities, families, citizens, clients, workers, service purchasers and providers that give meaning and content to responsibilisation. It is applied and resisted "here and now" in constantly changing contexts and encounters. Therefore, it is reasonable to examine the realisation of responsibilisation at the grass-roots level as it is talked into being and made sensible in everyday interaction and as the lived experiences of the stakeholders at the margins of welfare services. When approaching responsibilisation from this bottom-up perspective, it is possible to make visible its conflicting meanings and consequences for everyday life and identities – and possible to study how the theoretical claims meet the "messiness", uncertainties and ambivalent realities of everyday life. As Barnett (2003: 35) and Goddard (2012: 349) remind us: the governmentality perspective and governance programmes are not stable, ready-made and finished. Instead they are experienced in many ways, they can be deviated from and modified, and there is always space for agency and resistance within local settings (see also Phoenix and Kelly 2013; Gradin Franzén 2015). Welfare clients and workers are thus not "puppets" that act according to top-down governance.

The governmentality literature brings forward significant analysis of the current society and welfare states in particular, and raises relevant issues about responsibilisation and more generally managing responsibilities among different stakeholders in society. So, this book owes a lot to this research tradition and uses its core findings on responsibilisation as important reflective grounds for empirical analyses. Yet, the governmentality literature and advanced liberalism offer only one particular interpretation and discourse of managing responsibilities. Trnka and Trundle (2014: 136) claim that "the term of 'responsibility' has been colonized in public life and political rhetoric by neoliberal discourses of responsibilisation", and continue by stating that there are other ways of understanding responsible subjects and responsibilisation (see also Beckmann 2013). For instance, citizens are bound to each other by "relations of care" and "social contract ideologies" in which the intent of actions is not based on the individual's own interests, wants and needs (on self-government) but on the well-being of others (Trnka and Trundle 2014). This book also pursues a search for the various dimensions of responsibilities and responsibilisation as follows: first, by concentrating on local-level practices, and second, by scrutinising them in relation to other societal concepts and discourses that consider managing responsibilities and becoming active citizens – namely empowerment and participation, consumerism and personalisation, recovery and resilience (e.g. Howell 2015). Since responsibilisation as it is defined in the governmentality literature is not the only discourse on managing responsibilities in society, it should be compared with other discourses that might challenge, change and modify the advanced liberal ways of governing communities, families, citizens, clients, workers, service purchasers and providers.

References

Anttonen, A. and Häikiö, L. (2011) "From social citizenship to active citizenship?", in J. Newman and E. Tonkens (eds) *Participation, Responsibility and Choice: Summoning the active citizen in Western European welfare states* (pp. 67–85), Amsterdam: Amsterdam University Press.

Asquith, N. (2009) "Positive ageing, neoliberalism and Australian sociology", *Journal of Sociology*, 45(3): 255–269.

Banks, S. (2004) *Ethics, Accountability and the Social Professions*, Basingstoke, UK: Palgrave Macmillan.

Barnett, N. (2003) "Local government, New Labour and 'active welfare': a case of 'self responsibilisation'?", *Public Policy and Administration*, 18(3): 25–38.

Barry, M. (2013) "Rational choice and responsibilisation in youth justice in Scotland: whose evidence matters in evidence-based policy?", *The Howard Journal of Criminal Justice*, 52 (4): 347–364.

Beck, U. (1992) *Risk Society: Towards a new modernity*, London: Sage.

Beck, U. (1999) *World Risk Society*, Cambridge: Cambridge University Press.

Beckmann, N. (2013) "Responding to medical crises: AIDS treatment, responsibilisation and the logic of choice", *Anthropology & Medicine*, 20(2): 160–174.

Bennett, J. (2008) "They hug hoodies, don't they? Responsibility, irresponsibility and responsibilisation in Conservative crime policy", *The Howard Journal of Criminal Justice*, 47(5): 451–469.

Berger, P.N. (2015) *ADHD som socialt og kulturelt fænomen: En analyse af, hvordan diagnosticerede dømte voksne og frontmedarbejdere med relation til Kriminalforsorgen tilskriver ADHD-diagnosen betydning* [ADHD as a Cultural and Social Phenomenon: An analysis of how diagnosed convicted adults and frontline workers associated with the Danish Prison and Probation Service attribute meaning to the ADHD diagnosis], Copenhagen: KORA & The Faculty of Social Sciences, Aalborg University.

Berger, P.N. and Eskelinen, L. (2016) "Negotiation of user identity and responsibility at a prerelease conference", *Qualitative Social Work*, 15(1): 86–102.

Bergmark, Å. (2001) "Den lokala välfärdsstaten? Decentraliseringstrender under 1990-talet" [Local welfare state? Decentralising trends in the 1990s], in *Välfärdsstjänster i omvandling* [Welfare services in transformation] (pp. 21–76), Stockholm: Fritzes, SOU 2001:52, retrieved 15 May 2016 from www.regeringen.se/rattsdokument/statens-offentliga-utredningar/2001/06/sou-200152/.

Broom, A., Meurk, C., Adams, J. and Sibbritt, D. (2014) "My health, my responsibility? Complementary medicine and self (health) care", *Journal of Sociology*, 50(4): 515–530.

Brown, B.J. and Baker, S. (2012) *Responsible Citizens: Individuals, health and policy under neoliberalism*, London: Anthem Press.

Brown, K.J. (2012) " 'It is not as easy as ABC': examining practitioners' views on using behavioural contracts to encourage young people to accept responsibility for their anti-social behavior", *Journal of Criminal Law*, 76(1): 53–70.

Brown, R.C.H. (2013) "Moral responsibility for (un)healthy behavior", *Journal of Medical Ethics*, 39(11): 695–698.

Buckingham, H. (2009) "Competition and contracts in the voluntary sector: exploring the implications for homelessness service providers in Southampton", *Policy and Politics*, 37(2): 235–254.

Butler, K. and Benoit, C. (2015) "Citizenship practices among youth who have experienced government care", *Canadian Journal of Sociology*, 40(1): 25–49.

Carney, T. (2008) "The mental health service crisis of neoliberalism: an Antipodean perspective", *International Journal of Law and Psychiatry*, 31(2): 101–105.

Clarke, J. (2005) "New Labour's citizens: activated, empowered, responsibilized, abandoned?", *Critical Social Policy*, 25(4): 447–463.

Colvin, C.J., Robins, S. and Leavens, J. (2010) "Grounding 'responsibilisation talk': masculinities, citizenship and HIV in Cape Town, South Africa", *The Journal of Development Studies*, 46(7): 1179–1195.

Cossman, B. (2007) *Sexual Citizens: The legal and cultural regulation of sex and belonging*, Palo Alto, CA: Stanford University Press.

Cossman, B. (2013) "Anxiety governance", *Law & Social Inquiry*, 38(3): 892–919.

Cradock, G. (2007) "The responsibility dance: creating neoliberal children", *Childhood*, 14(2): 153–172.

Dahlstedt, M. and Fejes, A. (2014) "Family makeover: coaching, confession and parental responsibilisation", *Pedagogy, Culture & Society*, 22(4): 169–188.

Dean, M. (1999) *Governmentality: Power and rule in modern society*, London: Sage.

Dent, M. (2006) "Patient choice and medicine in health care: responsibilization, governance and proto-professionalization", *Public Management Review*, 8(3): 449–462.

Feeley, M. and Simon, J. (1992) "The new penology: notes on the emerging strategy of corrections and its implications", *Criminology*, 30(4): 449–474.

Ferguson, I. (2007) "Increasing user choice or privatizing risk? The antinomies of personalization", *British Journal of Social Work*, 37(3): 387–403.

Fischer, J. and Neale, J. (2008) "Involving drug users in treatment decisions: an exploration of potential problems", *Drugs, Education, Prevention, and Policy*, 15(2): 161–175.

Foucault, M. (1977) *Discipline and Punish: The birth of the prison*, Middlesex: Penguin.

Foucault, M. (1982) "The subject and power", in L. Dreyfus and P. Rabinow (eds) *Michel Foucault: Beyond Structuralism and Hermeneutics* (pp. 208–226), Brighton: Harvester.

Foucault, M. (1988) "Technologies of the self", in L.H. Martin, H. Gutman and P.H. Hutton (eds) *Technologies of the Self: A Seminar with Michel Foucault* (pp. 16–49), London: Tavistock.

Foucault, M. (1991) "Governmentality", in G. Burchell, C. Gordon and P. Miller (eds) *The Foucault Effect: Studies in Governmental Rationality* (pp. 87–104), London: Harvester Wheatsheaf.

Foucault, M. (1997) *Ethics: Subjectivity and truth. Essential works of Michel Foucault 1954–1984*, Vol. 1, edited by P. Rabinow, New York: New Press.

Garsten, C. and Jacobsson, K. (2013) "Sorting people in and out: the plasticity of the categories of employability, work capacity and disability as technologies of government", *Ephemera: Theory & Politics in Organization*, 13(4): 825–850.

Goddard, T. (2012) "Post-welfarist risk managers? Risk, crime prevention and the responsibilization of community-based organizations", *Theoretical Criminology*, 16(3): 347–363.

Gradin Franzén, A. (2015) "Responsibilization and discipline: subject positioning at a youth detention home", *Journal of Contemporary Ethnography*, 44(3): 251–279.

Gray, G.C. (2009) "The responsibilization strategy of health and safety: neo-liberalism and the reconfiguration of individual responsibility for risk", *The British Journal of Criminology*, 49(3): 326–342.

Hansen Löfstrand, C. (2012a) "Homelessness as politics and market", in B. Larsson, M. Letell and H. Thörn (eds) *Transformations of the Swedish Welfare State: From social engineering to governance?* (pp. 247–261), Basingstoke, UK: Palgrave Macmillan.

Hansen Löfstrand, C. (2012b) "Homelessness as an incurable condition? The medicalization of the homeless in the Swedish special housing provision", in L. L'Abate (ed.) *Mental Illnesses: Evaluation, treatments and implications* (pp. 105–126). InTech, DOI: 10.5772/29533.

Healy, K. (2009) "A case of mistaken identity: the social welfare professions and New Public Management", *Journal of Sociology*, 45(4): 401–418.

Hodgson, D. (2001) "'Empowering customers through education' or governing without government?", in A. Sturdy, I. Grugulis and H. Willmott (eds) *Customer Service: Empowerment and entrapment* (pp. 117–134), London: Palgrave.

Houdt, F. and Schinkel, W. (2014) "Crime, citizenship and community: neoliberal communitarian images of governmentality", *Sociological Review*, 62(1): 47–67.

Howell, A. (2015) "Resilience as enhancement: governmentality and political economy beyond 'responsibilisation'", *Politics*, 35(1): 67–71.

Hörnqvist, Magnus (2001) *Allas vårt ansvar i praktiken: en statligt organiserad folkrörelse mot brott* [Everyone is on our responsibility: a governmentally organised citizen movement against criminality]. Stockholm: Kriminologiska institutionen, Stockholms universitet.

Ilcan, S. (2009) "Privatizing responsibility: public sector reform under neoliberal government", *Canadian Review of Sociology*, 46(3): 207–234.

Ilcan, S. and Basok, T. (2004) "Community government: voluntary agencies, social justice, and the responsibilization of citizens", *Citizenship Studies*, 8(2): 129–144.

Jayasuriya, K. (2002) "The new contractualism: neo-liberal or democratic?", *Political Quarterly*, 73(3): 309–320.

Juhila, K. and Günther, K. (2013) "Kunnan, järjestöjen ja asiakkaiden oikeudet ja velvollisuudet tilaaja-tuottajamallissa: tutkimus asumispalvelujen tarjouspyyntöasiakirjoista" [Rights and responsibilities of municipalities, non-governmental organizations and service users in the purchaser–provider model], *Janus*, 21(3): 298–313.

Juhila, K., Günther, K. and Raitakari, S. (2015) "Negotiating mental health rehabilitation plans: joint future talk and clashing time talk in professional client interaction", *Time & Society*, 24(1): 5–26.

Keddie, A. (2015) "New modalities of state power: neoliberal responsibilisation and the work of academy chains", *International Journal of Inclusive Education*, 19(11): 1190–1205.

Kemshall, H. (2002) "Effective practice in probation: an example of 'advanced liberal' responsibilisation?", *The Howard Journal of Criminal Justice*, 41(1): 41–58.

Kemshall, H. (2008) "Risks, rights and justice: understanding and responding to youth risk", *Youth Justice*, 8(1): 21–37.

Kolthoff, E., Huberts, L. and van den Heuvel, H. (2007) "The ethics of New Public Management: is integrity at stake?", *Public Administration Quarterly*, Winter: 399–439.

Lacey, A. and Ilcan, S. (2006) "Voluntary labor, responsible citizenship, and international NGOs", *International Journal of Comparative Sociology*, 47(1): 34–53.

Lantz, S. and Marston, G. (2012) "Policy, citizenship and governance: the case of disability and employment policy in Australia", *Disability & Society*, 27(6): 853–867.

Le Bianic, T. (2011) "Certified expertise and professional responsibility in organisations: the case of mental health practice in prisons", *The Sociological Review*, 59(4): 803–827.

Lemke, T. (2001) "The birth of bio-politics: Michel Foucault's lecture at the College de France on neo-liberal governmentality", *Economy and Society*, 30(2): 190–207.

Liebenberg, L., Ungar, M. and Ikeda, J. (2015) "Neo-liberalism and responsibilisation in the discourse of social service workers", *British Journal of Social Work*, 45(3), 1006–1021.

Lister, M. (2015) "Citizens, doing it for themselves? The Big Society and government through community", *Parliamentary Affairs*, 68(2): 352–370.

Lynch, M. (2000) "Rehabilitation as rhetoric: the ideal reformation in contemporary parole discourse and practices", *Punishment & Society*, 2(1): 40–65.

Lyon-Callo, V. (2000) "Medicalizing homelessness: the production of self-blame and self-governing within homeless shelters", *Medical Anthropology Quarterly*, 14(3): 328–345.

MacKinnon, D. and Derickson, K.D. (2013) "From resilience to resourcefulness: a critique of resilience policy and activism", *Progress in Human Geography*, 37(2): 253–270.

Martin, L.L. and Kettner, P.M. (1997) "Performance measurement: the new accountability", *Administration in Social Work*, 21(1): 17–29.

Matarese, M. (2009) "Help me help you: reciprocal responsibility in caseworker-client interaction in a New York City shelter", paper presented at *DANASWAC conference*, Gent, 20 August 2009.

May, J., Cloke, P. and Johnsen, S. (2005) "Re-phasing neoliberalism: New Labour and Britain's crisis of street homelessness", *Antipode: A Critical Journal of Geography*, 37(4): 703–730.

Michailakis, D. and Schirmer, W. (2010) "Agents of their health? How the Swedish welfare state introduces expectations of individual responsibility", *Sociology of Health and Illness*, 32(6): 930–947.

Miller, P. and Rose, N. (2008) *Governing the Present: Administering economic, social and personal life*, Cambridge: Polity Press.

Mueller-Hirth, N. (2012) "If you don't count, you don't count: monitoring and evaluation in South Africa NGOs", *Development and Change*, 43(3): 649–670.

Muncie, J. (2006) "Governing young people: coherence and contradiction in contemporary youth justice", *Critical Social Policy*, 26(4): 770–793.

Newman, J. and Tonkens, E. (2011) "Introduction", in J. Newman and E. Tonkens (eds) *Participation, Responsibility and Choice: Summoning the active citizen in Western European welfare states* (pp. 9–28), Amsterdam: Amsterdam University Press.

Numerato, D., Salvatore, D. and Fattore, G. (2012) "The impact of management on medical professionalism: a review", *Sociology of Health and Illness*, 34(4): 626–644.

O'Malley, P. (2009) "Responsibilization", in A. Wakefield and J. Fleming (eds) *The SAGE Dictionary of Policing* (pp. 277–279), London: Sage.

Osbourne, D. and Gaebler, J. (1993) *Reinventing Government: How the entrepreneurial spirit is transforming the public sector*, New York: Plume.

Parton, N. (2006) *Safeguarding Childhood: Early intervention and surveillance in a late modern society*, Basingstoke, UK: Palgrave Macmillan.

Pathak, P. (2013) "From New Labour to New Conservatism: the changing dynamics of citizenship as self-government", *Citizenship Studies*, 17(1): 61–75.

Peeters, R. (2013) "Responsibilisation on government's terms: new welfare and the governance of responsibility and solidarity", *Social Policy and Society*, 12(4): 583–595.

Phoenix, J. and Kelly, L. (2013) "'You have to do it yourself': responsibilization in youth justice and young people's situated knowledge of youth justice practice", *British Journal of Criminology*, 53(3): 419–437.

Pollack, S. (2010) "Labelling clients 'risky': social work and the neo-liberal welfare state", *British Journal of Social Work*, 40(4): 1263–1278.

Power, M. (1997) *The Audit Society: Rituals of verification*, Oxford: Clarendon.

Raitakari, S., Haahtela, R. and Juhila, K. (2015) "Tackling community integration in mental health home visit integration in Finland", *Health and Social Care in the Community*, DOI: 10.1111/hsc.12246.

Ramon, S. (2008) "Neoliberalism and its implications for mental health in the UK", *International Journal of Law and Psychiatry*, 31(2): 116–125.

Rasmussen, J. (2011) "Enabling selves to conduct themselves safely: safety committee discourse as governmentality in practice", *Human Relations*, 64(3): 459–478.

Roberts, C. (2006) "'What can I do to help myself?' Somatic individuality and contemporary hormonal bodies", *Science Studies*, 19(2): 54–76.

Rose, N. (1990) *Governing the Soul: The shaping of the private self*, London: Routledge.

Rose, N. (1999) *Powers of Freedom: Reframing political thought*, Cambridge: Cambridge University Press.

Rose, N. (2000) "Government and control", *The British Journal of Criminology*, 40(2): 321–339.

Rose, N. and Miller, P. (1992) "Political Power beyond the State: problematics of government", *British Journal of Sociology*, 43(2): 173–205.

Rose, N., O'Malley, P. and Valverde, M. (2006) "Governmentality", *Annual Review on Law and Social Science*, 2: 83–104.

Saario, S. (2014) *Audit Techniques in Mental Health: Practitioners' responses to electronic health records and service purchasing agreements*, Tampere: Acta Universitatis Tamperensis, 1907.

Saario, S. and Raitakari, S. (2010) "Contractual audit and mental health rehabilitation: a study of formulating effectiveness in a Finnish supported housing unit", *International Journal of Social Welfare*, 19(3): 321–329.

Saario, S. and Stepney, P. (2009) "Managerial audit and community mental health: a study of rationalizing practices in Finnish psychiatric outpatient clinics", *European Journal of Social Work*, 12(1): 41–56.

Sahlin, I. (2004) "Central state and homelessness policies in Sweden: new ways of governing", *International Journal of Housing Policy*, 4(3): 345–367.

Satka, M., Alanen, L., Harrikari, T. and Pekkarinen, E. (2011) "Johdatus lasten ja nuorten hallinnan kysymyksiin" [Introduction to the governmentality of children and youth], in M. Satka, L. Alanen, T. Harrikari and E. Pekkarinen (eds) *Lapset, nuoret ja muuttuva hallinta* [Children, youth and changing governance] (pp. 11–28), Tampere: Vastapaino.

Scoular, J. and O'Neill, M. (2007) "Regulating prostitution: social inclusion, responsibilization and the politics of prostitution reform", *British Journal of Criminology*, 47(5): 764–778.

Shamir, R. (2008) The age of responsibilization: on market-embedded morality, *Economy and Society*, 37(1): 1–19.

Share, M. and Strain, M. (2008) "Making schools and young people responsible: a critical analysis of Ireland's obesity strategy", *Health & Social Care in the Community*, 16(3): 234–243.

Silverstein, M. and Spark, R. (2007) "Social bridges falling down: reconstructing a 'troublesome population' of battered women through individual responsibilization strategies", *Critical Criminology*, 15(4): 327–342.

Solberg, J. (2011) "Accepted and resisted: the client's responsibility for making proposals in activation encounters", *Text & Talk*, 31(6): 733–752.

Stonehouse, D., Threlkeld, G. and Farmer, J. (2015) "'Housing risk' and the neoliberal discourse of responsibilisation in Victoria", *Critical Social Policy*, 35(3): 393–413.

Teghtsoonian, K. (2009) "Depression and mental health in neoliberal times: a critical analysis of policy and discourse", *Social Science and Medicine*, 69(1): 28–35.

Thörn, H. and Larsson, B. (2012) "Conclusions: re-engineering the Swedish welfare state", in B. Larsson, M. Letell and H. Thörn (eds) *Transformations of the Swedish Welfare State: From social engineering to governance?* (pp. 262–282), Basingstoke, UK: Palgrave Macmillan.

Tonkens, E. (2011) "The embrace of responsibility", in J. Newman and E. Tonkens (eds) *Participation, Responsibility and Choice: Summoning the active citizen in Western European welfare states* (pp. 45–65), Amsterdam: Amsterdam University Press.

Treloar, R. and Funk, L. (2008) "Mothers' health, responsibilization and choice in family care work after separation/divorce", *Canadian Journal of Public Health*, 99 (Supplement 2): S33–S37.

Trnka, S. (2014) "Domestic experiments: familial regimes of coping with childhood asthma in New Zealand", *Medical Anthropology*, 33(6): 546–560.

Trnka, S. and Trundle, C. (2014) "Competing responsibilities: moving beyond neoliberal responsibilisation", *Anthropological Forum: A Journal of Social Anthropology and Comparative Sociology*, 24(2): 136–153.

Trydegård, G.-B. (2001) "Välfärdstjänster till salu: privatisering och alternativa driftsformer under 1990-talet" [Welfare services on sale: privatisation and alternative directions in 1990s], in SOU 2001:52 *Välfärdsstjänster i omvandling* [Welfare services in transformation] (pp. 77–179), Stockholm: Fritzes, SOU 2001:52, retrieved 15 May 2016 from www.regeringen.se/rattsdokument/statens-offentliga-utredningar/2001/06/sou-200152/.

van der Land, M. (2014) "Citizens policing citizens: are citizen watches manifestations of contemporary responsible citizenship?", *Citizenship Studies*, 18 (3/4): 423–434.

Whiteford, M. (2010) "Hot tea, dry toast and the responsibilisation of homeless people", *Social Policy and Society*, 9(2): 193–205.

3 Responsibilities and current welfare discourses

*Kirsi Juhila, Suvi Raitakari and
Cecilia Hansen Löfstrand*

Introduction

Responsibilities and responsibilisation are among the core topics in current socio-political discussions on the transformation and new directions of Western welfare states, although the latter term is not necessarily used in this context. They are also strongly present in the professional conversations and social policy literature concerning the expected roles of workers and clients in the welfare services. This chapter focuses on these discussions and the related scholarly work that form and analyse influential welfare discourses. These discourses, along with the governmentality literature, are potentially important when developing further a theoretical and empirical understanding of the issue of responsibilisation (see Chapter 2).

The welfare discourses introduced in this chapter are based on "keywords" in the sense that Ferguson (2007; see also Clarke *et al.* 2007: 27) understands them when he refers to Williams' (1976) book *Keywords – A Vocabulary of Culture and Society*. Keywords, such as "participation" and "empowerment", carry multiple meanings and can be used in contradictory ways in different settings. The meanings related to them are positive and hard to resist (Ferguson 2007: 387–388). Furthermore, they are used in justifying certain directions of change that are argued to be inevitable in the current welfare states and services. These features make keywords powerful and applicable both in policy level argumentation and in the everyday welfare practices. They can belong to the vocabulary of service user movements promoting full citizenship for everyone, of social and health care professionals describing how they support and help their clients, or of managers and politicians seeking new ways to organise services or reduce costs. Also, researchers promote and reflect the keywords in making sense of the current welfare systems, welfare work and the realities of clients.

We will concentrate on the influential welfare discourses, and their underlying keywords, that (re)organise responsibilities between clients, workers, communities and the state. We do not make a thorough review of the roots or of the multiple meanings of the discourses. Instead, we will concentrate on how the discourses bring forward and problematise responsibilities between different stakeholders, particularly between clients and welfare workers in public services.

We have grouped closely related keywords together so that, altogether, six of them form three pairs of keywords, each pair representing a larger cluster of discourses. Each cluster has certain common features. The clusters are: (1) participation and empowerment discourses, (2) consumerism and personalisation discourses and (3) recovery and resilience discourses. Despite this grouping, the discourses are also interconnected and often refer to each other in the literature.

Participation and empowerment discourses

Participation

Participation is a valued premise in democratic societies, and it implies "citizen power" (Arnstein 1969). It is linked closely to the idea of active citizenship. In the general sense, participation means "being involved or associated with others in some activity" (André 2012). "Being involved" might take many forms and occur in diverse contexts: from joining in spontaneous demonstrations to voting in public referendums, or from influencing personal service matters to taking part in collective user movements, or from doing voluntary work in different civil society arenas to helping old relatives or neighbours in their daily lives. Despite the various forms and contexts, participation generally means an aim to influence something and make a difference: to create more sustainable or equal societies; to influence plans and decisions concerning one's own communities, neighbourhoods or services; or to increase one's own well-being or that of other people in need. Daremo and Haglund (2008: 132) write that "participation can be explained using the concept of engagement, which means to take part, to be involved, to be included, to be accepted and to have access to necessary resources". Having responsibility, being given responsibility and learning to take responsibility for one's life is seen as vital in promoting participation (Daremo and Haglund 2008; Kvarnström *et al.* 2013).

Participation is regarded both as an action of intrinsic value in democratic societies, and as a means of meeting and solving societal and individual challenges and problems. It is a principle that is hard to resist, because it is commonly understood as being absolutely good for everyone's well-being (Arnstein 1969: 216). It is expected that everyone, in the end, wants to participate and be active – and benefits from it.

In addition to the civil society context, participation is a strongly emphasised principle in social and health care services across Western societies (Beresford 2002; Kvarnström 2011; Kvarnström *et al.* 2012; Kvarnström *et al.* 2013; Matthies and Uggerhoej 2014; Raitakari *et al.* 2015). Client participation and service user involvement are intensively discussed and researched topics in social and health policies, and in services such as social work, mental health and nursing. An expectation has arisen from a variety of directions that clients should have more active roles and power regarding their own well-being and services (Pilgrim and Waldron 1998; Drake *et al.* 2010). National policy documents and legislation have globally articulated the importance of client participation and service user involvement. Service users, as well as welfare and health professionals in various settings, have promoted the principle of client participation (Cahill 1996; Collins *et al.* 2007; Browne and Hemsley 2008; Kvarnström 2011: 8; Kvarnström *et al.* 2012). The service user movement has played a significant role in highlighting user involvement as a human rights issue (e.g. Bassman 1997; Cook and Jonikas 2002).

Client participation is commonly understood in terms of both individual and collective participation. At the individual level, it is considered important that service users are provided with information and that they are active in setting goals, defining support measures and making choices regarding their personal services. At the collective level, it is emphasised that, as an important stakeholder group, service users should be involved in the planning, providing, assessing and researching of services (Lammers and Happell 2003; Beresford 2002; Kvarnström 2011; Raitakari *et al.* 2015).

Participation is regarded as an important right: something that citizens and clients are entitled to. Professionals and welfare workers are seen as responsible for encouraging, enabling and supporting them to use this right. However, in many cases there are serious difficulties in realising participation in health and social services. These might be related to the complex needs of clients, the attitudes of professionals, the dynamics of client–worker interaction, the ways services are designed and provided, and to structural factors affecting the delivery and receiving of welfare services (Hickey and Kipping 1998; Tobin *et al.* 2002; Fischer and Neale 2008). It is also argued that individuals should have the right not to become involved or to participate. Since service users have different interests and expectations about their possibilities and abilities to participate, there needs to be an option to choose to be non-active (Hickey and Kipping 1998; Lammers and Happell 2003: 387; Fischer and Neale 2008; Raitakari *et al.* 2015). Yet, these kinds of rights-based arguments can be marginalised if participation is increasingly understood as everyone's responsibility. When emphasising the responsibility of citizens and clients to participate, it is not understood as an individual's free choice, but as a duty of citizenship to overcome exclusion and welfare dependency (Jayasuriya 2002; Paddison *et al.* 2008).

The concept of participation is related to the notion of empowerment that we introduce next. As Kvarnström *et al.* (2013: 288) put it: "a person can be empowered by enhancement of the person's participation, or have the need of being empowered to be able to participate" (see also Beresford 2002: 95–96; Adams 2008; Paddison *et al.* 2008).

Empowerment

"Empowerment" is not a new keyword. It has been used and applied widely, for example, during the last four decades in community psychology and in social work (e.g. Rappaport 1987; Lee 2001; Lee and Hudson 2011). Adams (2008: xvi) defines empowerment as the capacity of individuals, groups, and/or communities to take control of their circumstances, exercise power and achieve their own goals, and the process by which, individually and collectively, they are able to help themselves and others to maximize the quality of their lives.

Empowerment thus comprises both individual-level and community-level dimensions. According to Rappaport (1987: 121–122), it "conveys both a psychological sense of personal control or influence and a concern with actual social influence, political power and legal rights", and "is a process, a mechanism by which people, organizations, and communities gain mastery over their affairs".

"Empowerment" has a dual meaning also in the sense that it refers both to the self-empowerment processes of individuals and communities and to the activities of various professionals aiming to encourage and support "powerless" people in the processes of becoming more powerful. "Empower" as a verb can be defined as making someone "stronger and more confident, especially in controlling their life and claiming their rights" (Oxford Dictionaries). Thus, in "need" of empowerment are people or groups of people, often called "marginalised people", "excluded citizens" or "stigmatised groups", who are claimed to not have control and power in their own lives and communities. In the empowering processes, they are expected to gradually become enabled to master and improve their personal lives and living conditions, and to get a voice and a capacity to resist inequalities produced by institutional practices and societal structures.

As with participation, empowerment underlines active citizenship including the rights and abilities of (marginalised and excluded) individuals and communities to control their own lives and to help themselves. Paddison *et al.* (2008: 131) note that responsible participation "requires welfare recipients to engage 'in the active management of their lives' and this is portrayed as 'empowerment'" (see also Jayasuriya 2002: 309). Self-help and self-management rhetoric is associated with the advanced liberal way of governing and with responsibilisation, for example, through the aims of creating self-governing citizens and communities, and through strengthening welfare clients' responsibility for their own lives (see Chapter 2). Rose (2000: 334) sees empowerment as follows:

> The beauty of empowerment is that it appears to reject the logics of patronizing dependency that infused earlier welfare modes of expertise. Subjects are to do work on themselves, not in the name of conformity, but to make them free.... Autonomy is now represented in terms of personal power and the capacity to accept responsibility – not to blame others but to recognize your own collusion in that which prevents you from being yourself, and in doing so, overcome it and achieve responsible autonomy and personal power.

Not surprisingly, the ambiguities of empowerment discourses have been criticised in social policy and social work literature (Pollack 2010). In an advanced liberal context, welfare workers are charged with the responsibility of empowering clients by "reworking their subjectivities" to foster independent and self-sufficient citizens skilled at managing their own lives. Empowerment is thus argued to focus on individual factors, and the goal is a "cognitive restructuring" of the individual, rather than community-level work and structural or systematic changes. For example, Pollack (2010: 1268) claims that "social exclusion is reconfigured to be 'a state of mind' amendable to cognitive restructuring and empowerment" (see also Gray 2009: 451–453).

Conclusion

As important as criticism from the governmentality point of view is, participation and empowerment discourses cannot be understood solely as technologies of client self-responsibilisation at the margins of welfare services. The discourses also emphasise that to be able to govern one's life and to take responsibility for it are essential elements of well-being and self-determination. The possibilities and responsibilities for taking part and being involved in communities and services are vital for a good quality of life. To be responsible, and to be the one given responsibility, are linked to a respected position in social relations and in society. A critical question is, do individuals have sufficient resources, possibilities and support to become empowered and active? Empowerment requires empowering circumstances. Thus, the focus of the discourses is not solely on individual citizens' responsibilisation towards better life management and awareness of the duties in regard to other members of society (on responsibility projects): it is also on the disempowering policies, organisations, services and communities that need to be transformed towards more empowering and inclusive environments. It is highlighted that citizens, clients and professionals should create partnerships to do this transformation work. In particular, the service user movement can be seen as an important political actor (i.e. a way of participating) in aiming to create better services based on the wants and wishes of clients.

Consumerism and personalisation discourses

Consumerism

Whilst the participation and empowerment discourses discuss citizenship in a broad sense, which includes community-level actions, the discourses related to consumerism in public services look more narrowly at citizens as individual choice-making service users in social and health care services. Clarke *et al.* (2007: 2, 16) describe the difference between the citizen as a political construct and as a consumer:

> It is the consent of the citizen that empowers the state; while the state provides and secures the conditions that enable citizens to lead their lives.... In

contrast, the consumer is located in economic relationships. S/he is engaged in economic transactions in the marketplace, exchanging money for com- modified goods and services.... The shift from citizen to consumer individ- ualises relationships to collective services and depoliticizes "choice" by subjecting the public domain to the logics or markets and management that constitute "choice" in the private/market domain.

As with participation and empowerment, consumerism has been widely studied and discussed in the literature concerning human services (e.g. Clarke *et al.* 2007; Ferguson 2007; Fotaki 2009; Needham 2009; Greve 2009; Simmons *et al.* 2009). It has been demonstrated how the promotion of user choice that reflects consumerism has been dominant in welfare societies in recent decades.

In addition to the shift towards the logics of markets, consumerism is seeking another, related (ideological) shift: a move from a claimed welfare dependency and professional control to more active service user roles with associated rights and responsibilities. The overall idea is that clients should have more autonomy and control over their lives, including possibilities of making choices regarding the services they receive. Choices then concern where, how, when and by whom ser- vices are to be delivered (Le Grand 2005: 201; Raitakari and Juhila 2013). The claim is that the preferences of service users, instead of expert-defined needs, should be the first priority in providing services (Needham 2009: 79). In this frame, service users are defined as consumers, who, as individual rational actors, know what they need, make decisions that maximise their preferences (Fotaki 2009: 88) and "express their views about services via complaints and feedback systems" (Barnes 2009: 231). Such approaches draw on rational choice theories (e.g. Le Grand 2007), which claim that people make decisions in their own inter- ests by comparing the benefits and costs of existing choices (Greener 2007: 260). The duty of professionals, for their part, is to consult, inform and guide service users to make the best possible choices.

Similarly to the discourses of participation and empowerment, the discourses of consumerism have been associated with advanced liberalism and neo- liberalism in critical literature (e.g. Cossman 2013). Rose (2000; Miller and Rose 2008) connects consumerism to the core idea of responsibilisation, which approaches citizens as "enterprising selves" who work for their own independ- ence and well-being, and along with increased possibilities, make choices and thus also carry the risks of their individual choices (cf. Clarke 2005; Kemshall 2008; Teghtsoonian 2009). A serious criticism directed at these premises of con- sumerism is the extent to which service users in real life act as rational calcula- tive actors. Rational choice-making theories have been criticised for ignoring the fact that people invariably make choices in relation to other people, to certain embodied practices and institutional settings, and to certain power relations, which makes a rigid consumerist approach inappropriate (Jayasuriya 2002: 310; Mol 2008; Hansen Löfstrand and Juhila 2012). Furthermore, clients with limited financial resources and complex needs at the margins of welfare services are usually not in a position to choose, for instance, which social or health organisation provides their services, or if they should turn to private or public services. The clients also often lack information about complicated service systems and the options available to them. Bolzan and Gale (2002: 365) even claim that "a consumerist framework clearly establishes the role of professionals as gatekeepers to resources. How and when needs should be met is determined by these gatekeepers".

In the end, consumerism cannot, as Barnes (2009: 231) argues, "encompass the depth and diversity of means through which people who use health and social care services seek to influence the social relations of welfare" (see also Bolzan and Gale 2002). Furthermore, it is not that much of a usable discourse in welfare services such as probation and prison work that are inherently based on the control and involuntariness of the clients.

Personalisation

"Personalisation" as a new keyword and a way of organising and providing public services only emerged and started gaining support in the late 2000s, starting in the UK (Glendinning *et al.* 2008; Leece and Leece 2011: 205–206; Needham 2011; Spicker 2013). It comprises many similar meanings, as does consumerism, in regard to the responsibilities of clients and workers, but extends the responsibilities and rights of clients further. Its roots are in the ideas of person-centred services.

Leadbeater's (2004) pamphlet *Personalisation through participation*, as well as his other writings, is often cited when describing the core ideas of personalisation (e.g. Ferguson 2007; Needham 2011; Beresford 2014; Gardner 2014). According to Ferguson (2007: 393), these ideas include better customer friendliness, and users having more say in how they navigate in service systems and how money targeted to their services is spent. An important difference when compared with consumerism is that, in addition to service users being regarded as choice-making consumers, they are treated as co-producers and co-designers of services, as well as solution inventors and decision makers in their own and their communities' matters and problems (Leadbeater 2004; Ferguson 2007: 393; Glendinning *et al.* 2008). As Leadbeater (2004: 20) writes: "'Deep' personalisation would give users a far greater role – and also far greater responsibilities – for designing solutions from the ground up". Needham (2011: 65) concludes that "personalization advocates have weaved together a range of supportive discourses, encompassing the dignity and autonomy of the individual, the power of consumer choice and the failure of bureau-professional welfare states".

The most well-known way to implement personalisation is probably through personal budgets targeted at citizens who are eligible for publicly funded support (Leece and Leece 2011: 206; Hamilton *et al.* 2016; Larsen *et al.* 2015). Personal budgets are seen to represent the high-level user autonomy and choice; users can design their budgets according to their wants, and make decisions on how and where to purchase the support and services they need. Instead of offering similar services for everyone, personal budgets are argued to make personally tailored service packages possible. This calls for major shifts in the culture, roles and responsibilities of front-line workers (Glendinning *et al.* 2008; Hitchen *et al.* 2015). Individually targeted budgets are also expected to produce savings in public service costs. It has been shown in recent research that clients may gain autonomy, independence and recovery from personal budget arrangements that shift power to them, thus giving them a greater role in assessing their own needs and in making choices regarding services (e.g. Rabiee *et al.* 2009; Coyle 2011; Hitchen *et al.* 2015; Larsen *et al.* 2015).

However, personalisation has been a target of a similar kind of criticism as consumerism. Since the emphasis of personalisation is on individual service tailoring, it has been claimed to be unsuccessful in engaging with structural issues, such as inequalities among people and inadequacies in social and health care services (Ferguson 2007: 395). The limited amount of available service options has been recognised as a major barrier in designing one's own service package according to one's own wants (Ferguson 2007: 396). In addition, users have to negotiate their service packages (based on care plans) with various social and health care professionals, who simultaneously also often assess their entitlement to various services. This kind of "personal assessment" conducted by professionals "implies that the professional, rather than the consumer, will make the decisions" (Spicker 2013: 1261). User choice can thus be restricted in personalised services; service users may exercise their freedom only within boundaries set by politicians and professionals. Sometimes the promotion of personal budgets might even decrease service options: for example, current service producers often disappear from the "market" for being "old-fashioned" due to a changing commissioning policy. For instance, Needham's (2014) study shows how day centres for elderly and disabled people are seen as being unfit for a personalised service system and a tight fiscal context.

Despite the restrictions described above, personalisation discourses still expect clients to be active in planning their own services and to be responsible for making the right service choices. Beresford (2014) argues that in some cases personal budgets have meant the client "having to take on all the responsibilities and risks of running a personal budget without adequate information, back-up or support". So, "doing it alone" is not necessarily an empowering solution. Significantly increasing individual responsibility for personal budget management can bring along stress and uncertainty and thus decrease the well-being of clients (Hamilton *et al.* 2016: 732). As Hitchen *et al.* (2015: 387) conclude, "concerns remain about people's ability to manage the additional responsibilities, especially when unwell". Related to this, personalisation has been claimed to increase the need for brokerages, especially in the complex care need cases that demand navigation between many health and social services. In these cases, brokerage is named as a critical element in the success of the personalisation (Scourfield 2010). Brokers (i.e. special experts) supporting clients in managing personal budgets might take different (conflicting) roles, such as becoming advocates of the choices of oppressed citizens, advisers of clients to make the right choices, or gatekeepers of limited resources and unrealistic choices (Scourfield 2010;

Leece and Leece 2011). Such worker roles as an adviser, controller and guardian are easily accompanied by deficient and stigmatised client categories – not being active, able and responsible enough to make independent service choices and manage the duties of a purchaser.

Conclusion

Even though the discourses of consumerism and personalisation have been criticised, the rights of citizens to make service choices and to have control in their lives are not questioned per se. Glendinning (2008: 459–461) writes that there are strong arguments for emphasising user choice. It is fundamental to achieving citizenship, social inclusion and independence. At best, user choice reduces power differences between care providers and receivers. The capacity to exercise choice and control over one's life can also be an important recovery outcome itself. According to Hamilton *et al.* (2016: 722), "reclaiming control in terms of relatively small decisions may provide useful steps towards rebuilding an agentic sense of self". These kinds of arguments are familiar in what Beresford (2002) calls a democratic service user involvement approach that is "often framed in a rights discourse" (Noorani 2013: 50). The democratic approach accomplished through collective user movement actions underlines people's self-advocacy and participation in having more say in their own lives, services and society (Beresford 2002: 97). Choice offers opportunities to select and plan one's own services in a given service frame, or to respond to official health and social care initiatives to evaluate and give feedback about available services. It also offers opportunities for citizens who have experiences of using social and health care services (experts-by-experience) to voice their perspectives on service options and their contents, and on more general issues of personal and social life (Barnes and Cotterell 2012: xx–xxi).

Recovery and resilience discourses

Recovery

Oxford Dictionaries define recovery as "a return to a normal state of health, mind, or strength". According to this definition, recovery is thus a process during which something that has been lost is got back. This common-sense understanding of recovery does not, however, include all the variations that are connected to the recovery discourses in the current discussions. "Recovery" is a multidimensional keyword that comprises micro- and macro-level components (Jacobson and Curtis 2000; Barrett *et al.* 2010; Hunt and Stein 2012; Pilgrim and McCranie 2013). It is used to describe processes and characteristics of individuals tackling and living in difficult life situations. According to Jacobson and Greenley (2001: 482),

> Recovery refers to both internal conditions experienced by persons who describe themselves as being in recovery – hope, healing, empowerment,

and connection – and external conditions that facilitate recovery – implementation of the principle of human rights, a positive culture of healing, and recovery-oriented services.

Along with the recovery discourse, a new message has emerged that people with severe conditions can have a meaningful life and hope for the future, and that they are entitled to the same human rights as all members of society (Brown *et al.* 2008: 24).

Recovery resonates and overlaps with the participation, empowerment, consumerism and personalisation discourses (e.g. Deegan 1996; Carpenter 2002: 90; Barrett *et al.* 2010; Brennaman and Lobo 2011; Hunt and Stein 2012). This can be read from Deegan's (1996) personal account that resists the passive category of mental health client:

> Those of us who have been diagnosed are not objects to be acted upon. We are fully human subjects who can act and in acting, change our situation. We are human beings and we can speak for ourselves. We have a voice and can learn to use it. We have the right to be heard and listened to. We can become self determining. We can take a stand toward what is distressing to us and need not be passive victims of an illness. We can become experts in our own journey of recovery.

Davidson and Roe (2007) make a distinction between "recovery from" and "recovery in" mental illness, which are more widely applicable in social and health issues. They define "recovery from" as a process where the person recovers from problematic health conditions so that the symptoms are ameliorated, and the person is more or less off medication and returns to a healthier state (Davidson and Roe 2007: 463). "Recovery in", meanwhile, "refers to the process of living one's life, pursuing one's personal hopes and aspirations, with dignity and autonomy, in the face of the on-going presence of an illness and/or vulnerability to relapse" (Davidson and Roe 2007: 464; see also Anthony 1993). It emphasises a person's own agency, control over their own life and inclusion in communities, but it also takes into account the need for support and care. Pilgrim (2008: 297) describes "recovery in" as a community-oriented approach that "emphasizes supportive and personally tailored skills training to enable the patient to stay out of hospital and to maximize their ability to socially integrate". Pilgrim (2008: 297) also adds the third recovery approach, "recovery from invalidation", which is based on a social model (familiar from disability studies) and on a new social movement resisting expert-led diagnoses and treatment and coercive services. Within this approach, recovery is defined as a release and a successful survival from stigma-producing, deviant categorisations (see also Carpenter 2002: 89). These different approaches to recovery are in conflict with each other, yet they also help to depict the diversity of recovery and can be seen as complementary dimensions (Roberts and Wolfson 2004; Piat *et al.* 2009; Brennaman and Lobo 2011: 657).

Despite the multiple approaches to recovery described above, the discourse is often used in a way that constructs the individuals themselves as subjects of responsibility. It is depicted as gaining a new insight, strength and sense of self, of taking personal responsibility for one's life and future (Deegan 1996; Carpenter 2002: 88–89; Roberts and Wolfson 2004; Pilgrim and McCranie 2013: 46–50). Roy and Buchanan (2016: 406, 409) write that the concept of recovery has "been hijacked and reconfigured by government" to hide "a wider government agenda of responsibilisation, the reduction of welfare budget and highly individuated conceptions of citizenship". The concept has been associated with an advanced liberal way of governing, especially from the point of view of self-responsibilisation. For instance, Scott and Wilson (2011), who have studied a recovery programme called *Wellness Recovery Action Planning* (WRAP) that is targeted at people with mental health problems, argue that the programme adopts neoliberal ideas of individual responsibility and reflexive subjectivity: it "constructs the prudent, responsible subject, who plans ahead, maintains control, is constantly engaged in self-surveillance and works incessantly to sustain a healthy lifestyle" (Scott and Wilson 2011: 41). An important skill to be developed is an ability to identify the risks that might cause unwell-being.

Another reading of the recovery discourses also recognises the roles and responsibilities of professionals, other citizens and societal structural factors in individual recovery processes (Carpenter 2002; Mancini *et al.* 2005; Roy and Buchanan 2016). Professionals and other people are expected to have "recovery competencies" and capabilities to foster recovery-friendly interaction and keep up hope in severe situations. In addition, it is their task to develop, in cooperation with service users and experts-by-experience, recovery-led working practices and services (e.g. Anthony 1993; Deegan 1996; Jacobson and Curtis 2000; Roberts and Wolfson 2004).

Critics of recovery discourses warn about being too optimistic for a speedy recovery and setting too-high expectations on individuals, because of the risks of disappointment, self-blame and "blaming the victims". Recovery optimism may mean that service users are not given the right and acceptance to be ill and helpless (Roberts and Wolfson 2004; Piat *et al.* 2009: 205). Others have pointed out that when the recovery discourses – as in contemporary society – are drawn on more broadly, outside of a medical context and by people other than doctors, for example in relation to societal problems such as homelessness, it might contribute to a medicalisation of the problem of homelessness (Lyon-Callo 2000; Hansen Löfstrand 2012). As concluded by Lyon-Callo (2000: 340–341), within the shelter industry, a medicalised discourse "produces everyday practices of self-disclosure and self-government as routine habits that are accepted as 'common sense' ".

Resilience

"Resilience" can be defined as "the capacity to recover quickly from difficulties; toughness" (Oxford Dictionaries). Resilience and recovery are thus related concepts that attract a diverse range of professionals, educators, researchers and policy makers. The keyword "resilience" is widely and increasingly used in relation to mental health problems, other illnesses and disabilities, but also among others related to traumas and psycho-social adversities, substance abuse, violence and child abuse, natural and man-made catastrophes, conflicts and warfare (Herrman *et al.* 2011; Walker and Cooper 2011; Bulley 2013; Simmons and Yoder 2013; Marriott *et al.* 2014; Kukihara *et al.* 2014; Sudmeier-Rieux 2014; Howell 2015). Essential themes in the literature are: What does it mean to be a resilient person? What enhances resilience? Who or what are responsible for it? (e.g. Herrman *et al.* 2011; Shastri 2013; Khanlou and Wray 2014).

Resilience, in a narrow sense, can be considered as a personal trait, strength and ability that helps individuals to survive within difficult life situations. Like Herrman *et al.* (2011: 259) put it: "The central question is how some girls, boys, women, and men withstand adversity without developing negative physical or mental health outcomes" (see also Marriott *et al.* 2014: 18; Peer and Hillman 2014: 93). Resilience is typically connected to such characteristics as "self-efficacy, perseverance, good social skills and good communication skills, together with the aforementioned supportive networks" (Fougere *et al.* 2012: 707).

There are also more broad and interactive ways to conceptualise resilience that concentrate on protective and supportive forces at societal, cultural, community, family and individual levels (Herrman *et al.* 2011; Marriott *et al.* 2014; Khanlou and Wray 2014). Collectives and communities as wholes may also be seen as able to recover and be resilient or be responsible for promoting the wellbeing of individuals (Bulley 2013; Khanlou and Wray 2014; Muir and Strnadová 2014). Cultural resilience is related to the persistence of socio-ecological systems and collective identities in the face of change and their ability to transform into more desirable states when required (Rotarangi and Stephenson 2014: 503; Folke 2006).

Welsh (2014) has constructed a comprehensive typology of resilience that comprises both narrow and wider definitions of the concept. He locates the origin of the concept in two parallel approaches, which he calls "socio-ecological" and "psycho-social" resilience. Both deal with the recovery capacities in the contexts of adverse events, disturbances and crises. Whilst the socio-ecological approach concentrates on larger environmental and human systems (Folke 2006), the latter one concentrates on individuals and their nearby communities (Welsh 2014: 16–17), and is thus applied more in the social and health care contexts. Psycho-social resilience is understood as "the ability to recover from trauma, and a capacity to persist or sustain health and psychological wellbeing in the face of continuing adversity" (Ungar *et al.* 2008; Zautra *et al.* 2010 cited in Welsh 2014: 17). Shastri's (2013) description of how the concept is understood in psychiatry follows the same line:

> resilience stands for one's capacity to recover from extremes of trauma and stress. It is attributes of some people who manage to endure and recover fully, despite suffering significant traumatic conditions of extreme

deprivation, serious threat, and major stress. Resilience in a person reflects a dynamic union of factors that encourages positive adaptation despite exposure to adverse life experiences.

In the resilience discourses, responsibilities to promote and generate toughness are distributed between the state, citizens, service users and professionals very much in a similar way as in the recovery discourses. Although both concepts usually concentrate on personal survival, healing and growth, they simultaneously perceive the importance of social context and social support in surviving in life.

Critical reading (increasingly popular according to Howell (2015: 67] of the resilience concept associates it with governmentality and argues that it implies a new way to govern based on individual and community responsibilisation; communities, families and individuals are made responsible for becoming resilient. For example, Welsh (2014: 19) writes about "the governmentalisation of resilience", by which he means that the resilient subjects are conceived as "responsible for transforming themselves in the face of a world of contingency whilst also increasing resistance to exogenous and internal shocks by limiting the potential of events to provoke change". There is the danger that a shift towards the resilience discourses bypasses root causes and power issues related to risks, disadvantages and vulnerabilities in societies (Bulley 2013; MacKinnon *et al.* 2013: 262–263; Rogers 2013; Sudmeier-Rieux 2014). For Rogers (2013: 322), "resilience is a form of governmentality that can have both positive and negative articulations". Negative articulations are based on state-centric, top-down knowledge and practices that govern from a distance, whereas positive articulations foster citizen participation and empowerment.

Conclusion

The critical readings of the discourses on recovery and resilience as governmental techniques are valuable, but the meanings of these ambiguous keywords are much more complex. As Rogers (2013: 322) puts it, there is a "tension between positive and negative forms of resilience as governmentality". The discourses carry emancipatory possibilities promoted, for example, by service user movements. Referring back to Davidson and Roe's (2007) and Pilgrim's (2008) definitions of different recovery approaches, "recovery in" and "recovery from" invalidation approaches emphasise the responsibilities of communities and societies (instead of recovering individuals) to accept differences among people and thus to deconstruct stigmatising categorisations and service practices. Similarly, resilience understood both as socio-ecological processes and psycho-social processes (Welsh 2014) helps to perceive recovery as interactional processes between individual and community responsibilities, and in this way it helps to resist the individualistic tones of governmentalisation and responsibilisation (Bottrell 2009; Rogers 2013). Furthermore, as Bottrell (2009) suggests, resilience need not be defined solely as a positive adaptation to circumstances and personal coping with adversity: individual or collective resistance against social and cultural inequalities should also be recognised as enabling, protective and justified forms of resilience that shift the emphasis from individual to social responsibilities. Harper and Speed (2012: 23) summarise the need to redefine the recovery and resilience discourses:

> We do not discount the need for recovery and resilience approaches to give a central importance to individual experience but it is absolutely vital that the conceptualization of individual experience is one that can be tied back to collective and structural experiences of distress, inequality and injustice.

Conclusion and discussion

In this chapter we have described influential welfare discourses by focusing on how the responsibilities of different stakeholders in welfare services are dealt with and reflected in them. To begin with, we grouped the discourses along with the keywords they are based on into three clusters: (1) participation and empowerment discourses, (2) consumerism and personalisation discourses and (3) recovery and resilience discourses.

All the discourses are interconnected, but the three clusters of discourses also differ from each other with their special emphases on the responsibilities between clients and welfare workers.

Participation and empowerment discourses operate primarily on a community and civil society level, and approach clients in an active citizenship frame. This means that service users are expected both to be involved in planning their own services and to take part in such collective, service user actions that aim to develop better welfare services and better service practices. This kind of participation – having a voice – is a way to empowerment that results in increasing control of one's own circumstances and quality of life. Consumerism and personalisation discourses are based on the market-level logic. Instead of voice, the emphasis is on individual choice and entrepreneurial activity. Clients are understood as rational consumers, who are expected to have the capabilities to make the right, personal service choices from among the available options, and to also carry the risks of the choices they make. The third cluster of discourses, which relies on the keywords "recovery" and "resilience", refers mainly to the psychosocial level. This means that the focus is on personal healing pathways and abilities to survive illnesses and problems. Service users are treated as recovering individuals, who are engaging in their own healing actively, self-reflexively and with a resilient attitude.

Although they operate at different levels, it is notable that all the discourses emphasise the personal responsibilities of clients: they have a responsibility to participate, to empower themselves, to make wise service choices and to promote their own recovery. This kind of individual responsibilisation matches well with the ideas of an advanced liberal way of governing and the related technologies of self-government. Furthermore, the discourses create responsibilities for workers to advance the responsibilisation of their clients by encouraging, supporting, advising and controlling. In this sense, welfare workers can also be regarded as involved and responsibilised – the ones to be thanked or criticised for the successes and failures of clients. This responsibilisation of both clients and workers aims to end a claimed welfare dependency, and to decrease professional power and paternalistic practices. The most successful welfare work manages to make itself unnecessary for clients, or at least it significantly decreases the need for support and care. In the cases of failures, the dependency of clients continues and is seen as chronic. This kind of responsibilisation embedded in the influential welfare discourses easily stigmatises, and it blames both the clients and workers tackling long-term conditions and difficulties that are an inevitable reality at the margins of welfare services.

Nevertheless, it would be oversimplifying to approach the discourses only in the light of individual responsibilisation and self-governmental technologies. In this chapter we have shown that the welfare discourses also include meanings that pay attention to structural issues and the social origins of individual adversities. Thus, the discourses conceptualise both individual and social responsibilities. This is most obvious in the participation and empowerment discourses, whose cornerstone is an idea of the strengthening relationship between individual citizens and society. However, the recovery and resilience discourses that mostly concentrate on individual responsibilities and progress also contain structurally and socially oriented meanings (e.g. Deegan 1996; Jacobson 2001; Jacobson and Greenley 2001; Pilgrim and McCranie 2013). Communities, societies and service systems are understood as playing important roles in individual recovery processes, and thus being responsible for these processes (cf. "recovery from invalidation", Pilgrim 2008). Each discourse comprises critical arguments towards emphasising solely individual conduct; without empowering societal circumstances, social justice and equality, truly available service options or recovery-facilitating communities, welfare services and financial resources, individuals cannot be expected to become empowered citizens, wise consumers or recovered persons. So it is not reasonable or fair to put responsibilities and blame on individuals if the society does not first fulfil its responsibility to create and sustain inclusive and equal circumstances. It can be argued that the welfare discourses support and justify the dual responsibility of welfare workers, which are to help individuals to overcome barriers and difficulties in life and to take part in changing social conditions. However, nowadays the welfare discourses are more and more on the service of clients' self-responsibilisation and individualization of social problems. There is the risk that "the social" fades away and becomes unseen (Haynes 1998; Ferguson 2008; Hanssen *et al.* 2015; Kleppe *et al.* 2015).

In the welfare discourses, responsibilities are always tied to rights. This is often forgotten in the critical analyses of the discourses. According to the discourses, individuals have not only responsibilities but also rights to participate, to make choices and to be treated as being capable of recovering. In this sense, the discourses construct clients as full citizens with accompanied rights. Furthermore, welfare workers are constructed as resources – to which clients are entitled – in gaining full and active citizenship. Looking from the clients' rights perspective, workers have responsibilities to encourage clients to participate and be active at all levels of society, to coach them in choice making, to inform them about available options and to support them in their recovery processes.

The keywords that we have examined in this chapter – "participation", "empowerment", "consumerism", "personalisation", "recovery" and "resilience" – carry positive connotations in the current discussions concerning the transformation of Western welfare systems in a way that enables the citizens to have more active and powerful roles in societal and personal lives. They are thus hard to resist. However, the keywords have been problematised in the critical literature, especially from the advanced liberal point of view; some usages of the keywords can produce negative consequences that are to be resisted, such as discrimination and victim blaming. Jayasuriya (2002) calls this dilemma of an empowering liberal aim that is also one of disempowering results as a "paradox of liberal intent and illiberal outcomes".

In the critical governmentality literature, influential welfare discourses are sometimes approached as "big policies" (Howell 2015: 68). Howell (2015: 68), who claims that resilience is increasingly associated to governmentality, writes that in this "big policies" approach, "to some extent, subjects then are treated as 'dupes' (and not, for instance, engaged in multiple contestations, shaping, or even taking pleasure in governance)". Since the keywords carry multiple meanings and are used for various purposes, resistance can be accomplished in challenging and strengthening certain meanings of them and downgrading others. If the keywords have been hijacked for certain governance purposes, such as distributing responsibilities solely to clients for quick recovery, they can be hijacked back for the original professional purposes, such as emphasising the role of social factors and social responsibilities in the well-being of citizens. It is also possible to create new meanings for the keywords, or even to invent new keywords if the current ones are too occupied with an advanced liberal understanding of responsibilisation. Whether and how these kinds of struggles and discourse shifts exist, and whether certain "big policies" are dominant in grassroots level welfare practices, are matters of empirical investigation. In the next chapter, we introduce methodological approaches and analytic concepts for this kind of empirical research.

References

Adams, R. (2008) *Empowerment, Participation and Social Work*, Fourth Edition, Basingstoke, UK: Palgrave Macmillan.

André, P. with the collaboration of Martin, P. and Lanmafankpotin, G. (2012) "Citizen Participation", in L. Côté and J.-F. Savard (eds) *Encyclopedic Dictionary of Public Administration*, retrieved 15 June 2016 from www.dictionnaire.enap.ca/Dictionnaire/en/home.aspx.

Anthony, W.A. (1993) "Recovery from mental illness: the guiding vision of the mental health service system in the 1990s", *Psychosocial Rehabilitation Journal*, 16(4): 11–24.

Arnstein, S. (1969) "A ladder of citizen participation in the USA", *Journal of the American Institute of Planners*, 35(4): 216–224.

Barnes. M. (2009) "Authoritative consumers or experts by experience: user groups in health and social care", in R. Simmons, M. Powell and I. Greener (eds) *The Consumer in Public Services: Choice, values and difference* (pp. 219–234), Bristol: Policy Press.

Barnes, M. and Cotterell, P. (2012) "Introduction: from margin to mainstream", in M. Barnes and P. Cotterell (eds), *Critical Perspectives on User Involvement* (pp. xv–xxvi), Bristol: Policy Press.

Barrett, B., Young, M.S., Teague, G.B., Winarski., J.T., Moore, K.A. and Ochshorn, E. (2010) "Recovery orientation of treatment, consumer empowerment, and satisfaction with services: a mediational model, *Psychiatric Rehabilitation Journal*, 34(2): 153–156.

Bassman, R. (1997) "The mental health system: experiences from both sides of the locked doors", *Professional Psychology: Research and Practice*, 28(3): 238–242.

Beresford, P. (2002) "User involvement in research and evaluation: liberation or regulation?", *Social Policy and Society*, 1(2): 95–105.

Beresford, P. (2014) *Personalisation*, Bristol: Policy Press, Kindle edition.

Bolzan, N. and Gale, F. (2002) "The citizenship of excluded groups: challenging the consumerist agenda", *Social Policy and Administration*, 36(4): 363–375.

Bottrell, D. (2009) "Understanding 'marginal' perspectives: towards a social theory of resilience", *Qualitative Social Work*, 8(3): 321–339.

Brennaman, L. and Lobo, M.L. (2011) "Recovery from serious mental illness: a concept analysis", *Issues in Mental Health Nursing*, 32(10): 654–663.

Brown, C., Rempier, M. and Hamera, E. (2008) "Correlates of insider and outsider conceptualizations of recovery", *Psychiatric Rehabilitation Journal*, 32(1): 23–31.

Browne, G. and Hemsley, M. (2008) "Consumer participation in mental health in Australia: what progress is being made?", *Australasian Psychiatry*, 16(6): 446–449.

Bulley, D. (2013) "Producing and governing community (through) resilience", *Politics*, 33(4): 265–275.

Cahill, Jo (1996) "Patient participation: a concept analysis", *Journal of Advanced Nursing*, 24(3): 561–571.

Carpenter, J. (2002) "Mental health recovery paradigm: implications for social work", *Health and Social Work*, 27(2): 86–99.

Clarke, J. (2005) "New Labour's citizens: activated, empowered, responsibilized, abandoned?", *Critical Social Policy*, 25(4): 447–463.

Clarke, J., Newman, J., Smith, N., Vidler, E. and Westmarland, L. (eds) (2007) *Creating Citizen-Consumers: Changing publics and changing public services*, London: Sage.

Collins, S., Britten, N., Ruusuvuori, J. and Thompson, A. (2007) "Understanding the process of patient participation", in S. Collins, N. Britten, J. Ruusuvuori and A. Thompson (eds) *Patient Participation in Health Care Consultations: Qualitative perspectives* (pp. 3–21), Berkshire: McGraw-Hill, Open University Press.

Cook, J.A. and Jonikas, J.A. (2002) "Self-determination among mental health consumer/survivors: using lessons from the past to guide the future", *Journal of Disability Policy Studies*, 13(2): 87–95.

Cossman, B. (2013) "Anxiety governance", *Law & Social Inquiry*, 38(3): 892–919.

Coyle, D. (2011) "Impact of person-centred thinking and personal budgets in mental health services: reporting a UK pilot", *Journal of Psychiatric and Mental Health Nursing*, 18(9): 796–803.

Daremo, Å. and Haglund, L. (2008) "Activity and participation in psychiatric institutional care", *Scandinavian Journal of Occupational Therapy*, 15(3): 131–142.

Davidson, L. and Roe, D. (2007) "Recovery from versus recovery in serious mental illness: one strategy for lessening confusion plaguing recovery", *Journal of Mental Health*, 16(4): 459–470.

Deegan, P.E. (1996) "Recovery as a journey of the heart", *Psychiatric Rehabilitation Journal*, 19(3): 91–97.

Drake, R.E., Deegan, P.E. and Rapp, C. (2010) "The promise of shared decision making in mental health", *Psychiatric Rehabilitation Journal*, 34(1): 7–13.

Ferguson, I. (2007) "Increasing user choice or privatizing risk? The antinomies of personalization", *British Journal of Social Work*, 37(3): 387–403.

Ferguson, I. (2008) *Reclaiming Social Work: Challenging neo-liberalism and promoting social justice*, London: Sage.

Fischer, J. and Neale, J. (2008) "Involving drug users in treatment decisions: an exploration of potential problems", *Drugs, Education, Prevention, and Policy*, 15(2): 161–175.

Folke, C. (2006) "Resilience: the emergence of a perspective for social-ecological systems analyses", *Global Environmental Change*, 16(3): 253–267.

Fotaki, M. (2009) "Are all consumers the same? Choice in health, social care and education in England and elsewhere", *Public Money and Management*, 29(2): 87–94.

Fougere, A., Daffern, M. and Thomas, S. (2012) "Toward an empirical conceptualisation of resilience in young adult offenders", *Journal of Forensic Psychiatry & Psychology*, 23(5/6): 706–721.

Gardner, A. (2014) *Personalisation in Social Work*, 2nd Edition, London: Sage.

Glendinning, C. (2008) "Increasing choice and control for older and disabled people: a critical review of new developments in England", *Social Policy and Administration*, 42(5): 451–469.

Glendinning, C., Challis, D., Fernandez, J.L., Jacobs, S., Jones, K., Knapp, M. and Wilberforce, M. (2008) *Evaluation of the Individual Budgets Pilot Programme: Final report*, retrieved 23 November 2015 from www.york.ac.uk/spru.

Gray, P. (2009) "The political economy of risk and the new governance of youth crime", *Punishment & Society*, 11(4): 443–458.

Greener, I. (2007) "Choice and voice: a review", *Social Policy and Society*, 7(2): 255–265.

Greve, B. (2009) "Can choice in welfare states be equitable?", *Social Policy and Administration*, 43(6): 543–556.

Hamilton, S., Tew, J., Szymczynska, P., Clewett, N., Manthorpe, J., Larsen, J. and Pinfold, V. (2016) "Power, choice and control: how do personal budgets affect the experiences of people with mental health problems and their relationships with social workers and other practitioners?", *British Journal of Social Work*, 46(3): 719–736.

Hansen Löfstrand, C. (2012) "Homelessness as an incurable condition? The medicalization of the homeless in the Swedish special housing provision", in L. L'Abate (ed.) *Mental Illnesses: Evaluation, treatments and implications* (pp. 105–126). InTech, DOI: 10.5772/29533.

Hansen Löfstrand, C. and Juhila, K. (2012) "The discourse of consumer choice in the Pathways Housing First Model", *European Journal of Homelessness*, 6(2):47–68.

Hanssen, J.K., Hutchinson, G.S., Lyngstad, R. and Sandvin, J.T. (2015) "What happens to the social in social work?", *Nordic Social Work Research*, 5(Supplement 1): 115–126.

Harper, D. and Speed, E. (2012) "Uncovering recovery: the resistible rise of recovery and resilience", *Studies in Social Justice*, 6(1): 9–25.

Haynes, K.S. (1998) "One hundred year debate: social reform versus individual treatment", *Social Work*, 43(6): 501–509.

Herrman, H., Stewart, D., Diaz-Granados, N., Berger, E.L., Jackson, B. and Yuen, T. (2011) "What is resilience?", *Canadian Journal of Psychiatry*, 56(5): 258–265.

Hickey, G. and Kipping, C. (1998) "Exploring the concept of user involvement in mental health through a participation continuum", *Journal of Clinical Nursing*, 7(1): 83–88.

Hitchen, S., Williamson, G.R. and Watkins, M. (2015) "Personal budgets for all? Implementing self-directed support in mental health services", *Action Research*, 13(4): 372–391.

Howell, A. (2015) "Resilience as enhancement: governmentality and political economy beyond 'responsibilisation'", *Politics*, 35(1): 67–71.

Hunt, M.G. and Stein, C.H. (2012) "Valued social roles and measuring mental health recovery: examining the structure of the tapestry", *Psychiatric Rehabilitation Journal*, 35(6): 441–446.

Jacobson, N. (2001) "Experiencing recovery: a dimensional analysis of recovery narratives", *Psychiatric Rehabilitation Journal*, 24(3): 248–256.

Jacobson, N. and Curtis, L. (2000) "Recovery as policy in mental health services: strategies emerging from the state", *Psychiatric Rehabilitation Journal*, 23(4): 333–341.

Jacobson, N. and Greenley, D. (2001) "What is recovery? A conceptual model and explication", *Psychiatric Services*, 52(4): 482–485.

Jayasuriya, K. (2002) "The new contractualism: neo-liberal or democratic?", *Political Quarterly*, 73(3): 309–320.

Kemshall, H. (2008) "Risks, rights and justice: understanding and responding to youth risk", *Youth Justice*, 8(1): 21–37.

Khanlou, N. and Wray, R. (2014) "A whole community approach toward child and youth resilience promotion: a review of resilience literature", *International Journal of Mental Health & Addiction*, 12(1): 64–79.

Kleppe, L.C., Heggen, K.M. and Engebretsen, E. (2015) "Dual ideals and single responsibilities: a critical analysis of social workers' responsibility for the ideal of promoting justice at the individual and the societal level", *Nordic Social Work Research*, 5(1): 5–19.

Kukihara, H., Yamawaki, N., Uchiyama, K., Arai, S. and Horikawa, E. (2014) "Trauma, depression, and resilience of earthquake/tsunami/nuclear disaster survivors of Hirono, Fukushima, Japan", *Psychiatry & Clinical Neurosciences*, 68(7): 524–533.

Kvarnström, S. (2011) *Collaboration in Health and Social Care: Service user participation and teamwork in interprofessional clinical microsystems*, Jönköping: School of Health Sciences, Dissertation Series 15.

Kvarnström, S., Hedberg, B. and Cedersund, E. (2013) "The dual faces of service user participation: implications for empowerment processes in interprofessional practice", *Journal of Social Work*, 13(3): 287–307.

Kvarnström, S., Willumsen, E., Andersson-Gäre, B. and Hedberg, B. (2012) "How service users perceive the concept of participation, specifically in interprofessional practice", *British Journal of Social Work*, 42(1): 129–146.

Lammers, J. and Happell, P. (2003) "Consumer participation in mental health services: looking from a consumer perspective", *Journal of Psychiatric and Mental Health Nursing*, 10(4): 385–392.

Larsen, J., Tew, J., Hamilton, S., Manthorpe, J., Pinfold, V., Szymczynska, P. and Clewett, N. (2015) "Outcomes from personal budgets in mental health: service users' experiences in three English local authorities", *Journal of Mental Health*, 24(4): 219–224.

Leadbeater, C. (2004) *Personalisation through Participation: A new script for public services*, Demos: London, retrieved 23 November 2015 from www.demos.co.uk/files/PersonalisationThroughParticipation.pdf.

Lee, J.A.B. (2001) *The Empowerment Approach to Social Work Practice: Building a beloved community*, New York: Columbia University Press.

Lee, J.A.B. and Hudson, R.E. (2011) "Empowerment approach to social work practice", in F.J. Turner (ed.) *Social Work Treatment: Interlocking theoretical approaches* (pp. 157–178), Oxford: Oxford University Press.

Leece, J. and Leece, D. (2011) "Personalisation: perceptions of the role of social work in a world of brokers and budgets", *British Journal of Social Work*, 41(2): 204–223.

Le Grand, J. (2005) "Inequality, choice and public services", in A. Giddens and P. Diamonds (eds) *The New Egalitarianism* (pp. 200–210), London: Policy Network.

Le Grand, J. (2007) *The Other Invisible Hand*, Princeton, NJ: Princeton University Press.

Lyon-Callo, V. (2000) "Medicalizing homelessness: the production of self-blame and self-governing within homeless shelters", *Medical Anthropology Quarterly*, 14(3): 328–345.

MacKinnon, D. and Derickson, K.D. (2013) "From resilience to resourcefulness: a critique of resilience policy and activism", *Progress in Human Geography*, 37(2): 253–270.

Mancini, M.A., Hardiman, E.R. and Lawson, H.A. (2005) "Making sense of it all: consumer providers' theories about factors facilitating and impeding recovery from psychiatric disabilities", *Psychiatric Rehabilitation Journal*, 29(1): 48–55.

Marriott, C., Hamilton-Giachritsis, C. and Harrop, C. (2014) "Factors promoting resilience following childhood sexual abuse: a structured, narrative review of the literature", *Child Abuse Review*, 23(1): 17–34.

Matthies, A.-L. and Uggerhoej, L. (eds) (2014) *Participation, Marginalisation and Welfare Services: Concepts, politics and practices across European countries*, Surrey: Ashgate.

Miller, P. and Rose, N. (2008) *Governing the Present: Administering economic, social and personal life*, Cambridge: Polity Press.

Mol, A. (2008) *The Logic of Care: Health and the problem of patient choice*, London: Routledge.

Muir, K. and Strnadová, I. (2014) "Whose responsibility? Resilience in families of children with developmental disabilities", Disability & Society, 29(6): 922–937.

Needham, C. (2009) "Editorial: consumerism in public services", *Public Money and Management*, 29(2): 79–81.

Needham, C. (2011) "Personalization: from story-line to practice", *Social Policy & Administration*, 45(1): 54–68.

Noorani, T. (2013) "Service user involvement, authority and the 'expert-by-experience' in mental health", *Journal of Political Power*, 6(1): 49–68.

Oxford Dictionaries: Language matters. www.oxforddictionaries.com.

Paddison, R., Docherty, I. and Goodlad, R. (2008) "Responsible participation and housing: restoring democratic theory to the scene", *Housing Studies*, 23(1): 129–147.

Peer, J.W. and Hillman, S.B. (2014) "Stress and resilience for parents of children with intellectual and developmental disabilities: a review of key factors and recommendations for practitioners, *Journal of Policy & Practice in Intellectual Disabilities*, 11(2): 92–98.

Piat, M., Sabetti, J., Couture, A., Sylvestre, J., Provencher, H., Botschner, J. and Stayner, D. (2009) "What does recovery mean for me? Perspectives of Canadian mental health consumers", *Psychiatric Rehabilitation Journal*, 32(3): 199–207.

Pilgrim, D. (2008) "'Recovery' and current mental health policy", *Chronic Illness*, 4(4): 295–304.

Pilgrim, D. and McCranie, A. (2013) *Recovery and Mental Health: A critical sociological account*, Basingstoke, UK: Palgrave Macmillan.

Pilgrim, D. and Waldron, L. (1998) "User involvement in mental health service development: how far can it go?", *Journal of Mental Health*, 7(1): 95–104.

Pollack, S. (2010) "Labelling clients 'risky': social work and the neo-liberal welfare state", *British Journal of Social Work*, 40(4): 1263–1278.

Rabiee, P., Moran, N. and Glendinning, C. (2009) "Individual budgets: lessons from early users' experiences", *British Journal of Social Work*, 39(5): 918–935.

Raitakari, S. and Juhila, K. (2013) "Kuluttajuusdiskurssit ja palveluvalinnat mielenterveyskuntoutuksen asiakaspalavereissa" [Consumer discourses and service choices in mental health rehabilitation meetings], in M. Laitinen and A. Niskala (eds) *Asiakkaat toimijoina sosiaalityössä* [Clients as agents in social work] (pp. 167–195), Tampere: Vastapaino.

Raitakari, S., Saario, S., Juhila, K. and Günther, K. (2015) "Client participation in mental health: shifting positions in decision-making", *Nordic Social Work Research*, 5(1): 35–49.

Rappaport, J. (1987) "Terms of empowerment/exemplars of prevention: toward a theory for community psychology", *American Journal of Community Psychology*, 12(2): 121–148.

Roberts, G. and Wolfson, P. (2004) "The re-discovery of recovery: open to all", *Advances in Psychiatric Treatment*, 10(1): 37–49.

Rogers, P. (2013) "Rethinking resilience: articulating community and the UK riots", *Politics*, 33(4): 322–333.

Rose, N. (2000) "Government and control", *The British Journal of Criminology*, 40(2): 321–339.

Rotarangi, S.J. and Stephenson, J. (2014) "Resilience pivots: stability and identity in a social-ecological-cultural system", *Ecology & Society*, 19(1): 502–511.

Roy, A. and Buchanan, J. (2016) "The paradoxes of recovery policy: exploring the impact of austerity and responsibilisation for the citizenship claims of people with drug problems", *Social Policy & Administration*, 50(3): 398–413.

Scott, A. and Wilson, L. (2011) "Valued identities and deficit identities: Wellness Recovery Action Planning and self-management in mental health", *Nursing Inquiry*, 18(1): 40–49.

Scourfield, P. (2010) "Going for brokerage: a task of 'independent support' or social work", *British Journal of Social Work*, 40(3): 858–877.

Shastri, P.C. (2013) "Resilience: building immunity in psychiatry", *Indian Journal of Psychiatry*, 55(3): 224–234.

Simmons, A. and Yoder, L. (2013) "Military resilience: a concept analysis", *Nursing Forum*, 48(1): 17–25.

Simmons, R., Powell, M. and Greener, I. (eds) (2009) *The Consumer in Public Services: Choice, values and difference*, Bristol: Policy Press.

Spicker, P. (2013) "Personalisation falls short", *British Journal of Social Work*, 43(7): 1259–1275.

Sudmeier-Rieux, K.I. (2014) "Resilience: an emerging paradigm of danger or of hope?", *Disaster Prevention & Management*, 23(1): 67–80.

Teghtsoonian, K. (2009) "Depression and mental health in neoliberal times: a critical analysis of policy and discourse", *Social Science and Medicine*, 69(1): 28–35.

Tobin, M., Chen, L. and Leathley, C. (2002) "Consumer participation in mental health: who wants it and why?", *Australian Health Review*, 25(3): 91–100.

Ungar, M., Brown, M., Liebenberg, L., Cheung, M. and Levine, K. (2008) "Distinguishing differences in pathways to resilience among Canadian youth", *Journal of Community Mental Health*, 27(1): 1–13.

Walker, J. and Cooper, M. (2011) "Genealogies of resilience: from systems ecology to the political economy of crisis adaptation", *Security Dialogue*, 42(2): 143–160.

Welsh, M. (2014) "Resilience and responsibility: governing uncertainty in a complex world", *The Geographical Journal*, 180(1): 15–26.

Williams, R. (1976) *Keywords: A vocabulary of culture and society*, Glasgow: Fontana.

Zautra, A.J., Hall, J. and Murray, K. (2010) "Resilience: a new definition of health for people and communities", in J.W. Reich, A.J. Zautra and J.S. Hall (eds) *Handbook of Adult Resilience* (pp. 3–34), New York: Guildford Press.

4 Analysing the management of responsibilities at the margins of welfare practices

Kirsi Juhila and Christopher Hall

Introduction

In this book our focus is on the practices of welfare margins from the point of view of responsibilities and especially responsibilisation. Concentration on practices connects our approach to the so-called practice turn in social and human sciences (Schatzki *et al.* 2001). This means that we understand practices as "arrays of human activity" that are "organized around shared practical understanding" (Schatzki 2001: 2). It also means that we abandon dualistic ways of thinking (e.g. macro-micro) and do not privilege one human domain, such as individual experiences or structures, over the others (Schatzki 2001: 1–4). Llewellyn and Hindmarsh (2010: 11) notice the theoretical and methodological pluralism in the practice literature. Their own work combines ethnomethodology and organisation studies, because "practice-based studies seem to share with ethnomethodology an interest in the fine details and normative character of ordinary work" (Llewellyn and Hindmarsh 2010: 11). Likewise, we apply ethnomethodological ideas in our analyses of the grass-roots level practices at the margins of welfare services.

The origins of ethnomethodology, including the term itself, are in Harold Garfinkel's (1967) innovative work. Ethnomethodology (EM) studies human actions and reasoning in ordinary everyday practices (Heritage 1984; Francis and Hester 2004). However, by concentrating on everyday human practices, EM cannot be rendered as micro-science as opposed to structurally oriented macro approaches. EM studies can focus attention on how "macro" social phenomena are brought to life in particular encounters (Coulter 2001: 33–34). In regard to the advanced liberal way of governing and current welfare discourses (see Chapters 2 and 3), this means examining whether and how these phenomena are present and talked into being in grass-roots level welfare practices: for example, in clients' and worker's talk about their own and others' roles and identities in services, or in interactions between clients and workers. The main interest is in people's own orientations and perceptions, rather than explaining their talk and actions, for instance, with abstract social structures or psychological models.

Studying grass-roots level everyday practices means concentrating on talk, text and interaction in situ. Talk and text are approached as actions that construct social realities, not as reports on "something out there". Interactional emphasis means that social realities are understood as human interaction accomplishments, which are produced and justified in relation to contextual settings that people recognise and to which they position themselves. Based on these premises, we take the data (e.g. interview talk and various institutional encounters) as the starting point in analysing the practices of responsibilisation. It is in these settings that responsibilisation is made true, supported, bypassed, resisted and challenged. This is what we call the "management of responsibilities at the margins of welfare services".

Under the ethnomethodology frame it is possible to draw on different research methods such as conversation analysis (CA), membership categorisation analysis (MCA) and various discourse analytic applications (DA). In this book, these methods are combined in the sense that we apply certain analytic concepts developed and used within CA, MCA and DA that are informed by ethnomethodological premises. The chosen concepts are those that facilitate detailed analyses on how responsibilities are managed at the margins of welfare practices. The concepts are: responsibilities and accountability, categorisation, boundary work, sequentiality, advice-giving, narrative and resistance. We draw especially on studies which make use of analytic concepts that examine institutional human service practices. Such studies have increased considerably during the last three decades, although there are not yet many studies that combine analytic concepts to examine policy-level discourses.

In the following, we introduce the ethnomethodologically informed practice approach that is applied in the subsequent empirical chapters that concentrate on analysing the management of responsibilities from various angles. First, we discuss how policies based on an advanced liberal way of governing and welfare discourses (see Chapters 2 and 3) can be examined as human accomplishments in welfare service practices. Second, we describe how the above mentioned analytic concepts can be used in examining the management of responsibilities and the (possible) presence and usages of advanced liberal policies and welfare discourses at the margins of welfare services. The chapter ends up presenting the institutional settings and data of the empirical chapters (Chapters 5–10).

Advanced liberal policies and welfare discourses in grass-roots level practices

The term "responsibilisation" has been connected in the governmentality literature to a major ideological shift towards advanced liberal (or neoliberalist) policy making in Western welfare states. The core of this shift is in an increasing emphasis on individual and community responsibilities rather than state responsibilities (see Chapter 2). In addition, responsibilisation has been discussed in relation to the widely supported and used welfare discourses, including keywords such as "participation", "empowerment", "consumerism", "personalisation", "recovery" and "resilience", although these discourses also contain meanings that challenge the advanced liberal way of understanding responsibilisation (see Chapter 3). Relying on the ideas of the practice turn in social and human sciences, we aim to break down the macro-micro division and approach current policies and welfare discourses from the point of view of people's orientations in grass-roots level practices. This means concentrating on their talk, text and interaction in situ. As Potter and Hepburn (2010: 50) put it: "The analysis offered will be microscopic, but not as a contrast to macro social science – rather it is microscopic as it aims to capture the level of detail and organisation that the parties themselves demonstrably find relevant".

Alasuutari (2009: 70; Alasuutari and Quadir 2014) uses the concept "domestication" in examining how "supranational policy models are introduced within a nation-state". The roots of the concept are in anthropology and in consumption studies, where it has been applied to analysing how people actively and creatively "tame" new elements into their everyday practices (Alasuutari 2009: 66–67; Morley and Silverstone 1990). Alasuutari (2009: 70–71) claims that actual implementations of new models at a national level are always culturally bound and involve compromises between different stakeholders and powerful agents. Advanced liberal policies and welfare discourses such as consumerism and personalisation are good examples of supranational policy models and globally travelling ideas (Harris *et al.* 2015) that are currently implemented and domesticated in culturally specific ways in national-level welfare policy programmes and legislation in many Western countries. In this book, our focus is not primarily on nation-level domestication (e.g. on translation of governmental programmes or law texts, or on political debates). Instead, we take a step further to grass-roots level service practices and examine how supranational policy models and travelling ideas are present, used and resisted ("tamed") at the margins of welfare – the place where welfare workers and clients encounter each other.

Nearly 40 years ago, in their influential books, Lipsky (1980) and Prottas (1979) named the social and health care workers who encounter clients face-to-face in various welfare institutions as "street-level bureaucrats". Both authors stress that in their capacity as institutional representatives, street-level bureaucrats mediate between institutions and citizens. They meet the citizens (or clients) face-to-face as a routine part of their job, and they participate in institutional decision making on what services to provide and how to respond to the issues that arise. Due to these face-to-face routines, street-level welfare workers are the ones who have access both to institutional rules and procedures and to clients' experiences, needs and demands. It is their responsibility to translate institutional policy into daily, situated practice at the grass-roots level. This gives them a powerful position, and has considerable impact on institutions' practices and decision making as well as on the lives of the citizens. Their critical role is to interpret and fulfil the ambitions of government policies and to channel different services to the citizens (Hjörne *et al.* 2010: 303).

We regard Lipsky's and Prottas's work on the role and power of street-level bureaucrats as an important starting point in analysing the domestication of advanced liberal policies and welfare discourses. Street-level welfare workers do not just translate or simply put into practice the policies given "from above" – for instance, from national governments. They also have the power to modify, transform and even resist these policies as the key actors between policies and citizens. This is what Lipsky (1980) calls "discretion" in the work of street-level bureaucrats. What we wish to add to Lipsky's and Prottas's ideas is that welfare clients have the capacity to modify, translate, transform and resist dominant policies as they encounter workers in institutions or as they narrate their experiences as clients. Workers and clients also collaborate in doing this domestication and "taming" at the margins of welfare services.

In analysing the domestication and "taming" of advanced liberal policies and welfare discourses, we apply the ethnomethodological premises that emphasise the importance of studying local, in situ practices and especially the participants' (workers' and/or clients') orientations to policies and discourses in these practices (Garfinkel 1967; Heritage 1984; Hester and Eglin 1997a; Francis and Hester 2004). As Maynard (1988: 317) notes, we cannot assume that externally based "macro" structures simply reproduce themselves and are relevant features in people's talk and interaction in situ. Instead, our interest is on "how issues associated with wider social structures and discourses can be located, observed and described within situated action" (Evaldsson 2005: 764; 2007: 381). In doing this we inevitably draw on such extra-situational knowledge we have of current trends in Western welfare societies. However, as we have this knowledge, we are careful in demonstrating when and how (if at all) workers and clients orient to the policies and discourses associated with responsibilisation (cf. Llewellyn and Hindmarsh 2010: 16). People are not thus treated as products of responsibilisation, with the focus instead being on their local actions (Solberg 2011: 735), or to put it more precisely, on how they manage responsibilities in grass-roots level practices. In the analysis, we make use of certain analytic concepts developed in CA, MCA and DA that build bridges between the policies and discourses of responsibilisation and the practices in situ.

Analytic concepts in studying the management of responsibilities

Mediating analytic concepts

Building bridges between the policies and discourses of responsibilisation and practices in situ does not mean we can locate responsibilisation by simply searching for this concept in the grass-roots level welfare talk, texts and interactions. Responsibilisation is a concept developed to describe advanced liberal trends in current welfare states, and thus is unlikely to appear in everyday language use by those whom it might concern. While our interest is on how responsibilities are talked into being and managed at the margins of welfare services, we must be cautious not to interpret certain local welfare service practices uncritically and reductively as signs of responsibilisation. To succeed in that, we need mediating, analytic concepts (based on EM) that enable us to examine people's orientations in situ that may indicate responsibilisation practices. In what follows, we present these analytic concepts and provide grounds for how they might relate to the policies and discourses of responsibilisation. We start with the most obvious concept – responsibility – which is already implied in the formulation "responsibilisation". All the other analytic concepts presented in this chapter are connected in some way to the management of responsibilities.

Responsibilities

Responsibility and its plural form, responsibilities, are common concepts in the literature informed by ethnomethodology. Responsibility is closely linked to EM's basic principle of approaching "social order as the ongoing achievement of members of society conceived as practical actors" (Hester and Eglin 1997b: 1). In producing social order and orienting to it, people simultaneously create and maintain normative cultural expectations about how they and others ought to behave in particular settings. Social order and moral order are thus embedded in each other in people's actions (Jayyusi 1991: 246–248). Jayyusi (1991: 234) writes that

> Garfinkel's distinct achievement, was to elucidate the normative grounding of social order, and to elucidate it not as a general theoretic viewpoint or formal principle, but in and through the details of the ongoing, irremediably situated productions of order in particular settings – the in situ local organisation of intelligibility, and its normative embeddedness in "background expectancies".

Analysing the management of responsibilities, i.e. studying how people explicitly or implicitly orient to various responsibilities and talk them into being, is a way to examine moral order in action. And furthermore, by examining in detail responsibilities "in action", we can make interpretations and draw conclusions on whether this action contains issues underlined in the governmentality literature, such as emphasising individual responsibilities in life planning, choice making and risk taking. In other words: are these issues present as background expectancies in text, talk and interactions at the margins of welfare services?

To consider responsibility as a focus for study requires a different orientation to the macro version of responsibilisation. Approaches influenced by EM do not make assumptions about practices having an intrinsic nature or being the product of certain processes. Instead, the aim is to study how practices and dilemmas are managed in everyday talk, text and interaction, and to make analytic notions emerging from the data. It is taken as a starting point that "responsibility" is a word with a number of connotations. Martin (2007: 21) notes:

> In a mundane form [responsibility] permeates our talk about our duties and obligations, our jobs and tasks, the things we are in charge of, the things we are accountable for. At times it feels full of moral import – being

responsible for the welfare of a child – at other times it is simply some mundane tasks we must carry out or be in charge of.

Martin (2007: 28) suggests that there are four basic senses of the concept: "responsibilities as duties, obligations, jobs and tasks"; "being responsible for someone and/or something"; examining "who or what is responsible for something that has happened"; and "doing something responsibly". As Martin notes, there is a "family resemblance" between these possible uses in that they provide opportunities for participants to manage situations by drawing on different features. In particular, the moral associations of responsibility are terrains to be negotiated. There are, therefore, opportunities in everyday practices to upgrade or downgrade possible accusations of being responsible or irresponsible, to negotiate who is responsible for what tasks and to assess which features indicate responsible conduct. That is why, in this book, responsibilities are dealt with as negotiable matters.

Responsibilities can be explored by drawing on some of the key analytic concepts informed by the ethnomethodological research orientation – accountability, categorisation, boundary work, interaction order, advice-giving, narrative and resistance – which we now move on to scrutinise.

Accountability

Accountability is a concept that is tied to social and moral order and thus also inherently connected to the concept of responsibility (Matarese and Caswell 2014: 47). Accountability means that people are held responsible – account-able – for their actions (Garfinkel 1967: 1). Accountability is present in all text, talk and interaction, but its contents and forms are context-bound: "Any setting organises its activities to make its properties as an organized environment as practical activities detectable, countable, recordable, tell-a-story-aboutable, analysable – in short, accountable" (Garfinkel 1967: 22). Institutional settings, such as the various welfare service settings that are the subject of this book, create specific environments for the management of responsibility and accountability. As Mäkitalo (2003: 496) puts it: "being responsible in institutional encounters thus implies being able to respond in accountable and comprehensible manners as we engage in them".

In welfare service interactions, workers' accountability (and responsibility) includes, for instance, giving well-justified advice and recommendations; and, for their part, clients' accountability (and responsibility) involves following workers' advice or explaining the reasons for not doing so. Accountability bound to (welfare) institutions is not limited only to the face-to-face encounters between workers and clients. For instance, audiences to whom workers are expected to display accountability also include service purchasers, managers, other welfare organisations and (tax-paying) citizens in general. Hence, accountability can be examined in textual reporting or documenting, multi-professional or multi-organisational meetings and public inquiries, or in interview talk.

Similarly, clients have various audiences. In the widest sense, the audience can be named as dominant cultural expectations: that which is expected from good citizens in a certain historical-societal era. For example, the current emphasis of individual responsibility and responsibilisation can be regarded as forming a part of general cultural expectations, which workers and clients attend to when accounting for their actions.

Examining accountability means concentrating on such occasions of text, talk and interaction where people provide reasons for their behaviour. Accountability becomes visible especially when people explain "the gap between action and expectation" (Scott and Lyman 1968: 46). Explaining the gap signals that one has not fulfilled the expected responsibilities, or that one has failed to meet them. Failures can be explained by justifying, excusing or blaming (Scott and Lyman 1968). In justifying, the actor does not admit that the real failure has happened, since behaviour has had certain positive outcomes or reasonable causes. Excuses are accounts "in which one admits that the act in question is bad, wrong, or inappropriate but denies full responsibility" (Scott and Lyman 1968: 47). Blaming, on the other hand, can be regarded as accounts in which troublesome behaviour is explained as being due to omissions or commissions for which the actors can be held responsible (cf. Pomerantz 1978; Hall *et al.*, 2006: 34; Juhila *et al.* 2010). Blame can be targeted at other people or at oneself (self-blame). Accounts signal how people treat both themselves and others as socially responsible or irresponsible actors. In this book, our interest is on the extent to which accountability and accounts facilitate and/or promote the ideas related to responsibilisation. For instance, do clients account for not being active or self-governed enough, or do workers account for not being able to be effective in preventing risks or producing "responsible citizens"?

Categorisation

Categorisation – our third analytic concept that originated in EM – is also closely tied to the concepts of responsibility and accountability. Matarese and Caswell (2014: 48) state that the constructing of others and ourselves "according to moral categories is a common by-product of accounts, particularly when the account is managing a transgression or a gap between expectation and action" (see also Scott and Lyman 1968). Sacks's work on membership categorisation is important here (Sacks 1972a, 1972b, 1992). He noted that "a great deal of the knowledge that members of a society have about the society is stored" in categories (Sacks 1992: 40–41). Jayyusi (1991: 240) describes Sacks' ideas on categories and their moral characteristics:

> Sacks' notion on category bound actions, rights, and obligations not only points out the moral features of our category concepts, but also provides thus for the very moral accountability of certain actions or omissions. His elucidation of the notion of certain categories as standardised relational pairs not only uncovers features of the organisation of members' conventional

knowledge of the social world, but clearly demonstrates, via his detailed empirical analysis, how that knowledge is both morally constituted and constitutive of moral praxis – it provides for a variety of ascriptions, discoveries, imputations, conclusions, judgement etc. on the part of mundane reasoners. It shows how our knowledge is constitutive of, and provides for, a *moral inferential logic* – a logic of moral inference that is at the same time a moral grounding of practical inference [italics in original].

A standardised relational pair (Sacks 1972a) refers to pairs of categories such as doctor–patient or parent–child where "it is known what the typical rights, obligations, activities, attributes and so forth are of the one part of the pair with respect to the other" (Francis and Hester 2004: 40). In studying welfare service practices, a worker–client pair is relevant. Another important pair in our book, although not so evident, is purchaser–provider. Commonly, we expect the members of particular categories to behave in a certain way and to have certain obligations and rights. For instance, when a client and a worker meet in a substance abuse treatment clinic, the worker's obligations and expected actions include mapping the client's problems with substance use, discussing them and then suggesting appropriate treatment and solutions. The client's role in turn includes disclosing and discussing possible problems and risks and responding to the worker's suggestions. If either of the pairs "breaks" these moral expectations, one's responsibilities in the setting and interaction, an explanation is often required. The worker might explain that the client is "not yet ready" (or unmotivated or irresponsible) for treatment and is therefore in the wrong place if s/he is not willing to talk about the problem and take steps towards recovery. Or the client might accuse the worker of being unprofessional and ineffective (or even lazy) or sick, as s/he seems to have no expertise or skills to offer remedies to the client's tricky situation. Hence, in accounting for behaviour that appears to break category-bound expectations, other moral categories are available to be evoked.

Cultural categorisations are not static. Cultural and moral expectations of the obligations, rights and activities that are bound to the categories of welfare clients and welfare workers are transformed, in particular those associated with the changes in wider welfare policies and discourses (see Chapters 2 and 3). For instance, these categories are likely to be transformed by the advanced liberal shift from social to individual responsibilities and the associated criticisms of welfare dependency and demands for more active citizenship. In addition, welfare discourses can have a similar effect. Participation and empowerment discourses emphasise clients' rights and abilities to control their own lives, as do ideas connected to personalisation, recovery and resilience. Clients nowadays are therefore expected most of all to be active and self-responsible. Furthermore, expectations concerning welfare workers have been re-examined in the era of managerialism. Their new category-bound characteristics include such attributes as effectiveness, marketing (especially in regard to service purchasers) and a customer service orientation.

However, whether, and how, the policies and discourses associated with responsibilisation have changed the category expectations of welfare clients and workers, and thus have been domesticated into street-level welfare practices, is an empirical matter. In studying local practices, we examine whether and how clients and workers orient to these policies and discourses and their possibly new category-bound expectations. In this book, we discover the ways in which people themselves make sense of wider social structures by categorising themselves or others (Hester and Eglin 1997a; Mäkitalo 2014). An important aspect in examining this is to pay attention to stigmatising and coercive categorisations. For example, do clients (and workers) compare themselves and their everyday lives to ideal models of active citizens and, while doing that, construct themselves as responsible selves or failures?

Boundary work

Boundary work, unlike our other analytic concepts, does not originate directly from the ethnomethodological research tradition. Gieryn (1983) first coined the term "boundary work" to denote how scientists distinguish their work from that of non-science (Slembrouck and Hall 2014: 62). The term has thereafter been applied especially in the studies concerning occupational jurisdiction and work boundaries (e.g. Abbott 1995; Allen 2000). Gieryn (1983: 781) emphasises that boundary work includes demarcation that "is routinely accomplished in practical, everyday settings". Similarly, Allen (2000: 351) writes that work boundaries are interactionally accomplished and profoundly situated. Accordingly, Wikström (2008: 60) defines boundary work as "the processes by which boundaries, demarcations or other divisions are constructed, negotiated, reinforced, or redefined". Hall and Slembrouck (2014; Hall *et al.* 2010) have developed the concept towards a more rigorous, ethnomethodologically informed analysis of everyday welfare service practices and interactions. They approach boundary work as ways in which "workers and clients manage the dilemmas of the personal, professional, organisational and cultural divisions during everyday encounters" (Slembrouck and Hall 2014: 62).

In this book, we understand boundary work as situated practices of professional (occupational) and organisational demarcation, including (re)negotiations of responsibilities between clients, workers, services providers and purchasers: who is or should be responsible for what? Professional demarcation means negotiations and struggles between professions, or between professions and "volunteers concerning the skills and jurisdiction over a particular domain of work" (Hall *et al.* 2010: 349). For example, does work among homeless people with mental health problems belong more to the expertise of social workers or psychiatric nurses, or is it the domain of volunteer workers? Organisational demarcation can be based on professional boundaries, but it also has other dimensions (Saario *et al.* 2015).

According to Hernes (2004: 10), "organization emerges through processes of drawing distinctions, and it persists through the reproduction of boundaries". At the margins of welfare services, distinctions might be made, for instance, between substance abuse treatment and mental health organisations, which are both multi-professional but which define their domain of work differently based on how problems are formulated. Municipal service purchasers and commissioners also often participate in negotiations dealing with welfare organisations' domains of work: which organisations are best fitted to take responsibility for which client groups?

Boundary work is categorisation in the sense that professions and organisations differentiate themselves (we) from others (they) by emphasising their particular expertise and responsibilities in relation to others. This kind of categorisation has been approached in the boundary work literature from the perspective of how professions construct specific expertise and monopolies by competing with other professions (Lamont and Molnár 2002: 178). Such competition involves both inclusionary and exclusionary boundary work: arguing that "this belongs to our expertise and domain of work, whilst that does not since it demands different kinds of skills". At the margins of welfare services, exclusionary boundary work is an important focus of research, as it might produce and categorise client groups that are not recognised as belonging to a specific expertise of any professions or organisations. In contrast, inclusionary boundary work means relying less on service allocation in terms of pre-set client categories and providing flexible services based on individual needs, which, for instance, "hold on" to clients in difficult life situations.

Boundary work is moral by nature as it deals with the question of allocating responsibility. For example, not fulfilling the responsibilities attached to certain professions and organisations creates the need for accounting for "failure" or exclusionary actions. Boundaries never disappear but are redrawn, reinforced and redefined (Hernes 2004: 11; Wikström 2008: 60). In this book, we aim to examine where, when and how boundaries between the state (municipalities), service providers, workers and citizens (clients) are (re)negotiated in an advanced liberal manner (see Chapter 2). Furthermore, if so, how is this negotiation recognisable in the grass-roots level practices of marginal welfare services? For instance, is boundary work used in a way that justifies greater client and citizen responsibilities? Or do increasing expectations of cost-effectiveness produce "unwanted" client groups and social problems, which professions or organisations easily (re)define from their expertise? Are those grass-roots level workers whose expertise and responsibilities are at stake able to do boundary work on their own terms, or is it strongly regulated by others (e.g. purchasers)?

Sequentiality

Sequentiality, another of Sacks's (1992) key findings, which means temporal ordering of turns of talk, is a useful analytic concept particularly when the focus of analysis is on naturally occurring institutional interaction at the margins of welfare services. The basis of sequentiality lies in the interaction order. Goffman (1983: 2) developed the idea of the interaction order to underline the importance of approaching face-to-face interaction as "a substantive domain of its own right" that is based on the rules of the interactional organisation itself. Heritage (2001: 48) writes that the interaction order "comprises a complex set of interactional rights and obligations, which are linked both to 'face' (a person's immediate claims about 'who s/he is' in an interaction), more enduring features of personal identity, and also to large-scale macro social institutions".

Interactional rights and obligations mean that certain shared norms of anticipated and jointly acceptable behaviour are present, and are used once individuals meet and talk to each other. Norms are thus both moral and relational. Violations of such norms are possible, but when individuals recognise violations as exceptions from the interaction order, they expect from others, or produce themselves, accounts for these violations. For instance, if you do not receive an answer from a person to whom you have asked a question, you might repeat the question. If you still do not get a response, you are entitled to start accounting for the missing answer – for example, you might wonder whether the question was not heard or was too difficult to respond to for the other person (Juhila *et al.* 2014b: 17–19).

Sequentiality is the cornerstone of the interaction order. Sacks "noticed that what speakers do in their next turns is related to what prior speakers do in the immediate prior turns" (Psathas 1995: 13). This relates to a "current speaker selects next" structure in which the speaker designs his/her words for a certain recipient, who then has a right and an obligation to respond (Sacks *et al.* 1974: 704). The recipients of the prior turns analyse information embedded in the turns, and display some interpretative conclusions of their own in the following turns of talk (Heritage and Atkinson 1984: 8). The basic structure of temporal sequentiality is called "adjacency pairs". Adjacency pairs are at least two turns long and have at least two parts (Psathas 1995: 18). One part always goes before the other, as in greeting–greeting, question–answer, suggestion–acceptance/ rejection, request–acceptance/rejection and complaint–excuse/justification pairs (Silverman 2007: 66). Adjacency pairs are both temporarily related (one part goes before the other) and "discriminatively" related (since the first part implicates what is the appropriate next part) (Psathas 1995: 18; Silverman 2007: 66–67). Participants in interaction expect questions to be answered or greetings to be responded to. The absences, or even short delays, of the second parts or "wrong" second parts are noticed and can be treated as indicators of some sort of interactional trouble (Psathas 1995: 18). Preference organisation is another important element of sequentiality. It means that the first turn sets up "normative expectations of what is to follow" (Antaki 2011: 2). This is linked to adjacency pairs: for instance, it is preferable to accept an invitation or a suggestion than to reject it. In the latter case (rejection) the second parts usually include some sort of account for the unexpected response.

Institutional interaction is based on the same universal norms of the interaction order and sequentiality as "ordinary" conversation and interaction. However, in institutional contexts, as in the organisations of marginal welfare services, interactional norms are also connected to the particular institutional tasks and allocation of roles. As Hindmarsh and Llewellyn (2010: 35) write, sequences can be used as a resource for work and can be applied in different organisational settings. For instance, care planning often includes form-based questions posed by a worker to a client, whose answers are then used as material in writing the final plan. A lack of answers produces difficulties in fulfilling the institutional task of care planning. The interaction order and sequentiality can therefore be seen to contain certain elements of responsibilisation in institutional interaction in the sense that both workers and clients are expected to behave as "responsible participants" in their face-to-face interaction (e.g. asking questions and answering them for care planning purposes, or providing accounts for not questioning or answering). In addition to the elements of responsibilisation embedded in the interaction order itself, sequentiality can be used for the special responsibilisation purposes. By this we mean that workers can target questions, suggestions, requests etc. on issues that are bound more explicitly to the wider policies and discourses of responsibilisation – for instance, "Have you visited the employment office since we last met?" or "I think you could take better care of your physical condition". In this book, we are particularly interested in the latter form of interactional responsibilisation, where the interaction order and sequentiality are used as devices in responsibilisation.

Advice-giving

Advice-giving is an integral part of worker–client interactions in all human services that seek to provide support, guidance, care and control for individuals in their everyday problems and life planning. Advice-giving has a future and change orientation. The content of advice indicates what clients are expected to do in order to solve problems or to achieve a better balance in their lives. Heritage and Sefi (1992: 368) define that in giving advice a worker "describes, recommends or otherwise forwards a preferred course of future action". Advice-giving is characteristically normative (Butler *et al.* 2010), as it creates certain expectations towards clients' future behaviour and also allocates responsibilities to fulfil these expectations. Advice-giving is therefore a clear example of producing moral order in action.

Advice-giving and receiving advice together form an adjacency pair, and are therefore part of the sequentially organised interaction order and embedded normative expectations. In worker–client interaction, advice-giving sequences are more often initiated by workers than by clients (Heritage and Sefi 1992; Silverman 1997; Vehviläinen 1999). Clients can sometimes seek advice directly by asking questions ("how should I make contact with the employment office?"), or indirectly, for instance, by disclosing their drinking problems. Worker-initiated advice-giving can also have various forms. Heritage and Sefi (1992) differentiate three forms:

- "overt recommendations" – for example, "well, my advice to you is that …";
- advice couched in the imperative mood – for example, "always be very very quiet at night";

- the use of verbs that express obligation – for example, "and I think you should involve your husband as much as possible" (Hall and Slembrouck 2014: 101).

The morally preferred response to professional advice-giving in worker–client interactions is to accept it and treat its content as valuable information with marked acknowledgement ("yes, I really should try to be more quiet"). However, more often responses are unmarked ("that's right", "mm"), which indicates that the advice does not offer new information, is unacknowledged or is even resisted (Heritage and Sefi 1992: 395–402).

As already mentioned, in this book we aim to demonstrate how sequentiality can be used as a tool, technique or strategy in conducting responsibilisation. Advice-giving and receiving sequences can be used in two senses. First, the contents of advice can indicate the direction of the preferred course of action that is seen as a "must" for clients to follow in order to become more independent and responsible citizens. Second, the ways in which clients receive advice can be interpreted (by workers) as signs of a responsible attitude they take towards advice and whether that attitude needs attention. However, these two dimensions in advice-giving – contents and forms of interaction – also might conflict. As Jefferson and Lee (1992: 531) suggest, "acceptance or rejection [of advice] may be in great part an interactional matter, produced by reference to the current talk, more or less independent of intention to use it, or actual subsequent use". So, a worker might be providing appropriate advice, but because of the style and timing of the formulation and the sequence of interaction in which it occurs, the advice is treated as interactionally inappropriate and is resisted or ignored by the client (Hall and Slembrouck 2014: 102).

Advice-giving and the contents of advice are connected to institutional tasks, organisational guidelines and contracts between service purchasers and providers, and more widely to prevailing policies and cultural expectations of citizen responsibilities and rights. Workers are therefore also "advised" to perform their work among clients in certain ways. If these "advisers" promote the ideas of responsibilisation, workers are pushed to give clients advice that is expected to support their independency and increase their self-helping and even self-advising capacities in future challenges and problems. Close analysis of advice-giving sequences in institutional interaction is required when examining whether and how this kind of domestication of responsibilisation policies and discourses occurs.

Narrative

Although it is more associated with literary studies, narrative theory and analysis is increasingly used across the social and human sciences, including ethnomethodologically oriented studies. Many features of social life are considered to be interpreted as, or constituted through, narrative, as speakers explain, illustrate or justify their talk through telling a story. Indeed, some authors suggest that it is our ability to make sense of our social world through storytelling that makes us human (e.g. Gubrium and Holstein 1998: 163; Jameson 1981: 13). To analyse everyday interaction, narrative approaches examine temporal aspects of talk and writing: how do speakers organise events in their talk? This is usually done with a beginning, middle and end that imply a move from one state of affairs to another, and in doing so, makes a point that has consequences for both narrator and listener/reader. As Riessman and Quinney (2005: 394) put it, "events are selected, organized, connected and evaluated as meaningful for a particular audience".

For the purposes of this book, two aspects of narrative analysis are particularly appropriate: narrative structure and performance. Narrative structure concentrates on how the story is organised – on the form rather than the content. Sacks (1992) analysed stories in conversation as one form of talk-in-interaction. As described in the section on sequentiality, a central feature of everyday conversation is its organisation in terms of turn-taking: speakers generally manage sequences of talk in terms, for example, of questions and answers, invitation and acceptance/rejection. To make space to tell a story in ongoing talk, the storyteller needs to create an agreement with the listener to talk for an extended period without interruption. This requires a "story preface", an announcement of an intention or request to tell a story: for example, "I must tell you what happened to me the other day". The listener is therefore constrained from interrupting until the story is completed with a closing comment such as "so that's what happened".

The most celebrated model for examining narrative structure is provided by the socio-linguist Labov (1972). He provides an ideal structure of a "fully formed narrative" based on the temporary organisation of the clauses in the speech. There are six elements:

- an abstract, which introduces the gist of the story to come;
- an orientation, which sets the scene;
- a complication, which introduces the problem or rupture in routine affairs;
- the evaluation, which indicates the significance of the event;
- the resolution, which deals with the problem;
- the coda, which rounds off the story.

Such a structure provides both causality and credibility to the story and is organised to counter what Labov calls the "so what" question. The evaluation in particular is a direct address to the audience that events happened in the way they did, and were (and are) important. Riessman (2008) uses the Labov model to understand how divorced people talk about relationship breakdown and make sense of their marital problems. She considers that the organisation of events in the stories and the significance given to them uncover displays of distress which would not have been possible through thematic analysis.

In contrast to studies of a narrative structure, research on narrative performance concentrates on the telling of the story. As Gubrium and Holstein (1998: 166) consider: "it casts storytelling as an ongoing process of composition rather than the more-or-less coherent reporting of experience". The evaluation clause in Labov's model implies an interruption in the temporality of the story, which directly addresses the audience. Interactive approaches examine ways in which stories are co-constructed, and their function in ongoing interaction. Storytelling is a practical activity produced for and with the listener – sometimes to entertain, sometimes to persuade. In particular, it aims to produce an authoritative construction of events and their significance, which is hard to challenge (see Rosulek 2010 on the closing arguments in court). As well as narratives told in everyday situations, research interviews can be approached as storytelling and story reception occasions.

Storytelling in ordinary (non-institutional) talk is likely to involve more complex methods of story preface and the negotiation of speaking turns. Conversational stories are rarely personal in the sense of belonging to a particular speaker, or bounded by formal structures. Instead, they are co-constructed, contested and constituted in relationships, often characterised by challenges, questions, clarifications and speculations (Ochs and Capps 2001). In institutional storytelling, the allocation of roles of narrator and listener is more likely to be established, with particular kinds of stories following partially predetermined storylines, in, for example, counselling, welfare offices and medical consultations. In court, narratives are restricted in the sense that the storyteller is encouraged to tell the temporary flow of the events but is prevented from indicating their significance. As Gubrium and Holstein (1998: 177) summarise: "narrative production is necessarily collaborative, even while it is institutionally informed".

In analysing the management of responsibilities, both aspects of narrative – structure and performance – are relevant. In regard to the organisation of the story, a crucial question is what kinds of roles and identities are allocated to different parties in the story: who are reported to be responsible for the complication of events, and who are given key roles in the resolution? Similar questions can be asked in examining how (client case) stories are co-constructed in client–worker interaction, in workers' team meetings, in interviews with clients and workers etc. Since responsibilities are managed and distributed in narratives, narratives can also include elements of responsibilisation: for example, who is to be blamed for problems (complications) that have emerged, and which party should change their behaviour in order to avoid problems in the future?

Resistance

Our last analytic concept is resistance, which we have already touched on in presenting other concepts. It is necessary to emphasise that policies and welfare discourses related to responsibilisation are not simply applied but also assessed, problematised and challenged in the practices of welfare services. Resistance can be practised by both parties – workers and clients – who are the subjects of responsibilisation at the margins of welfare services (see Chapter 2).

Practices of resistance can be approached from different angles (Juhila *et al.* 2014a). In institutional interactions, such as in worker–client conversations, multi-professional case-planning meetings or discussions between service purchasers and providers, resistance might be displayed in sequential actions. For example, clients are silent or produce only minimal responses to workers' inquiries during their job-seeking activities (passive resistance). They might question directly the meaning of these "hopeless" endeavours, make alternative suggestions regarding how to plan and organise their lives outside of the labour market, or display overall misalignment to the institutional purposes of encounters (e.g. Zimmerman 1998; MacMartin 2008; Broadhurst *et al.* 2012; Caswell *et al.* 2013). Workers, for their part, can resist, for instance, clients' suggestions concerning alternative ideas by challenging their rationality or responding passively. Similar kinds of sequential resistance can be present in other institutional interactions: for example, in discussing who is responsible for which occupational activities (boundary work), between workers representing different welfare organisations and/or professions, between managers and workers, between purchasers and providers, etc.

Another angle from which to approach resistance is to analyse it in relation to the categorisations that are engaged in the policies and discourses of responsibilisation. These policies and discourses carry certain kinds of moral expectations on different stakeholders' characteristics and responsibilities. For example, both workers and clients are expected to be active and productive; "failing" these expectations creates accountability. These kinds of categorisations are talked into being but also challenged in the practices of welfare services. In particular, categorisations that carry stigma and threaten individuals' faces (such as being non-active or not trying) (Goffman 1961, 1964) are often resisted by, for instance, denying one's membership in a category, by displaying one's own ordinariness or decency or by directly fighting back against stigmas (e.g. Juhila 2004; Osvaldsson 2004; Virokannas 2011). It is notable that categorisations can also be resisted on behalf of another party – for instance, a worker can defend a client who has been labelled as incapable by other welfare organisations.

The third orientation to this analytic concept is resistance that is targeted directly towards macro-level advanced liberal policies that promote the ideas of responsibilisation. For instance, the aims of activation policies or productivity programmes can be criticised as unrealistic, and thus their demands are seen as impossible to fulfil for workers and clients. This kind of criticism can be presented by all stakeholders individually in various settings at welfare services, and also by allying with each other.

Settings and data used in the book

As described above, in studying whether and how advanced liberal policies and welfare discourses on responsibilisation are present at the margins of welfare services, we focus on everyday practices. To examine these practices, we need to locate our studies in certain institutional settings. The main settings of the book are supported housing and floating support services organised by four non-governmental organisations (NGOs) for people with mental health problems and sometimes also with substance abuse problems. Two of the services have combined housing and services together (clients live in the accommodation sub-let by the NGO). Two have separated services and housing, and are therefore based more on support provided in clients' individually rented (or sometimes owner-occupied) flats. All are community-based services that are distinct, for example, from nursing homes; clients are expected to live quite independently without 24/7 support. The services can also be described as half-way services in the sense that clients quite often have histories of living in nursing homes or treatment periods in psychiatric hospitals, and in the future they are expected to become more independent. These services are thus not meant to be permanent solutions, but only temporary support in clients' recovery processes. From the point of view of responsibilisation, these half-way services can thus be seen to have a task to empower clients towards more self-responsible lives.

Although the services are run by NGOs, they are dependent on governmental and municipal funding. NGOs provide supported housing and floating support services based on a purchaser–provider model, meaning that the services are regularly tendered and managed according to a contract between a provider and a purchaser. In regard to responsibilisation, a split between providers and purchasers means that NGOs are expected to monitor, fulfil and report, for example, certain recovery outcomes (such as, after three years' support, clients are expected to move towards lighter support) that are stipulated in a contract. These kinds of expectations responsibilise grass-roots level workers to achieve the agreed performance indicators and recovery outcomes.

In addition to supported housing and floating services, we have data from three other institutional settings. So altogether our data settings include:

- four supported housing and floating support services;
- a project offering housing and social skills training for young adults with diagnosed schizophrenia;
- a low-threshold outpatient clinic for people with severe drug abuse problems;
- a prison and probation service.

The latter three are also run by NGOs with a contract based on a purchaser–providers spilt, which creates certain outcome expectations for grass-roots level work. In an overall local service system, they are situated at a lower level than half-way services; if clients' recovery processes (and responsibilisation) are assessed to have been progressing well, their next step could be, for instance, entitlement to some supported housing or floating support service.

A common feature of all the services is that they are targeted at adults who are defined as having complex needs. The "label" of having complex needs indicates that clients using these particular housing and support services often use other social and health services as well. So, there is quite a lot of negotiation and boundary work going on among organisations and professions: who are responsible for taking care of these multiple needs, and how are obligations divided between the responsible parties? However, it seems to us that the services, and particularly their grass-roots workers, carry a large (almost limitless) amount of responsibility for caring for, supporting and controlling their clients (cf. Brodwin 2013: 67). This is because they have regular, sometimes daily, contacts with the clients and their everyday struggles. The clients also recognise that this close relationship contains contradictory elements of trust, care, surveillance and control. This everyday closeness provides intimate and sometimes tense encounters to analyse how responsibilities are managed between the workers and the clients, and how these two parties understand their responsibilities in regard to other, more distant stakeholders.

Two of the supported housing and floating support services, the project for young adults and the low-threshold outpatient clinic are located in a big city in Finland. The other two supported housing and floating support services are situated in a large city in England, and the prison and probation service in a large Danish city. Finland and the United Kingdom (UK) differ somewhat from each other in regard to their (so far) prevailing welfare regimes: Finland (along with Denmark) represents a Nordic, social-democratic welfare state regime that is based on universal citizenship rights to social transfers, benefits and services, instead of relying on markets or communities (families) as primary sources of social security. The UK, in contrast, is closer to a liberal regime with more means-tested transfers, benefits and services (Esping-Andersen 1990). Furthermore, the UK and Finland are claimed to be at different phases in the implementation of advanced liberal governance. The UK can be regarded as a forerunner and Finland more like a follower in this sense (Koskiaho 2008). However, as Miller and Rose (2008: 212) argue, advanced liberal ideas have been promoted in all Western political regimes during recent decades (see Chapter 2). Because of this "international travelling" from country to country (e.g. Harris *et al.* 2015), we assume that the findings of this book are not relevant only in Finnish and English grass-roots level responsibilisation practices. Obviously, travelling ideas are always domesticated in certain national and local (organisational) contexts, but the analyses presented in this book can provide comparative and reflective grounds for forthcoming grass-roots level studies in different countries and welfare service contexts.

In demonstrating the management of responsibilities in the subsequent chapters, we make use of multiple sources of data. In addition, the contributors to the book have carried out ethnographic observations in the welfare services in order to perceive and understand better the local service settings and their general modes of operation. The data sources include:

1   interviews with clients, clients' care coordinators, grass-roots level and managerial level workers in the service-providing NGOs, and the commissioners as representatives of the service purchasers;
2   focus groups with the grass-roots workers in the services;
3   client–worker conversations during home visits;
4   multi-party case-planning meetings and conferences;
5   team meetings among the grass-roots level workers.

Interviews and focus groups were organised for the purposes of the study, while the other three types of data naturally occur in the sense that they are part of the everyday routines of the services. Each data type is explained in the following chapters in enough detail for the analysis to be understood. In collecting and analysing the data, the researchers have complied with ethical principles of research in human and social sciences in Finland and the UK. All data extracts have been anonymised. Although the data contain both researcher-invited and naturally occurring material, we approach all data as interactional conversations between the parties (e.g. between workers and clients, or interviewers and interviewees), where responsibilities and the elements of responsibilisation are discussed, negotiated and managed in various ways (cf. Potter 2002).

Conclusion and discussion

We have shown in this chapter how the concept of responsibilisation, which has been developed from a macro perspective, can be examined in grass-roots level everyday practices. This is done by drawing on analytic concepts developed in ethnomethodology or inspired by an ethnomethodological research orientation, as these enable a series of empirical studies of how responsibilities are constructed, performed and resisted in a variety of encounters at the margins of welfare services. Concepts such as accountability, categorisation and boundary work are available to be deployed by workers, clients and managers in a wide range of encounters and texts in order to facilitate the allocation and management of responsibilities. The analytic concepts serve as a toolbox in Chapters 5–10. Some of them – responsibility, accountability and resistance – are applied in every chapter, whereas others – categorisation, boundary work, sequentiality, advice-giving and narrative – are used more selectively depending on the main perspectives of the chapters. Likewise, the type of data analysed in each chapter varies depending on the perspective.

Failing to address adequately the management of responsibilities can result in strong accusations, disputes and negative characterisations. In particular, it is important to examine in detail how everyday welfare practices are premised upon wider policies and discourses related to responsibilisation, or to what degree there are opportunities for discretion, improvisation and resistance. Are there other discourses, drawing on, for example, welfare discourses such as participation, empowerment and recovery, that are available to challenge advanced liberal concepts associated with responsibilisation (see Chapter 3)?

References

Abbott, A. (1995) "Boundaries of social work or social work of boundaries?", *Social Service Review*, 69(4): 545–562.

Alasuutari, P. (2009) "The domestication of worldwide policy models", *Ethnologia Europaea*, 39(1): 66–71.

Alasuutari, P. and Quadir, A. (eds) (2014) *National Policy Making: Domestication of global trends*, Oxon and New York: Routledge.

Allen, D. (2000) "Doing occupational demarcation: the 'boundary work' of nurse managers in a district general hospital", *Journal of Contemporary Ethnography*, 29(3): 326–356.

Antaki, C. (2011) "Six kinds of applied conversation analysis", in C. Antaki (ed.) *Applied Conversation Analysis: Intervention and change in institutional talk* (pp. 1–14), Basingstoke, UK: Palgrave Macmillan.

Broadhurst, K., Holt, K. and Doherty, L. (2012) "Accomplishing parental engagement in child protection practice? A qualitative analysis of parent-professional interaction in pre-proceedings work under the Public Law Online", *Qualitative Social Work*, 11(5): 517–534.

Brodwin, P.E. (2013) *Everyday Ethics: Voices from the frontline of community psychiatry*, Berkeley: University of California Press.

Butler, C.W., Potter, J., Danby, S., Emmison, M. and Hepburn, A. (2010) "Advice implicative interrogatives: building 'client-centred support' in a children's helpline", *Social Psychology Quarterly*, 73(3): 265–287.

Caswell, D., Eskelinen, L. and Olesen, S.P. (2013) "Identity work and client resistance underneath of canopy of active employment policy", *Qualitative Social Work*, 12(1): 8–23.

Coulter, J. (2001) "Human practices and the observability of the 'macro-social'", in T.R. Schatzki, K. Knorr Cetina and E. von Savigny (eds) *The Practice Turn in Contemporary Theory* (pp. 29–41), London: Routledge.

Esping-Andersen, G. (1990) *The Three Worlds of Welfare Capitalism*, Cambridge: Polity Press.

Evaldsson, A.-C. (2005) "Staging insults and mobilizing categorizations in a multiethnic peer group", *Discourse & Society*, 16(6): 763–786.

Evaldsson, A.-C. (2007) "Accounting for friendship: moral ordering and category membership in preadolescent girls' relational talk", *Research on Language and Social Interaction*, 40(4): 377–404.

Francis, D. and Hester, S. (2004) *An Invitation to Ethnomethodology: Language, society and interaction*, London: Sage.

Garfinkel, H. (1967) *Studies in Ethnomethodology*, Cambridge: Polity Press.

Gieryn, T.F. (1983) "Boundary work and the demarcation of science from non-science: strains and interests in the professional ideologies of scientists", *American Sociological Review*, 48(6): 781–795.

Goffman, E. (1961, reprinted in 1991) *Asylums: Essays on the social situation of mental patients and other inmates*, London: Penguin Books.

Goffman, E. (1964, reprinted in 1990) *Stigma: Notes on the management of spoiled identity*, London: Penguin Books.

Goffman, E. (1983) "The interaction order", *American Sociological Review*, 48(1): 1–17.

Gubrium, J. and Holstein, J. (1998) "Narrative practice and the coherence of personal stories", *The Sociological Quarterly*, 39(1): 163–187.

Hall, C. and Slembrouck, S. (2014) "Advice-giving", in C. Hall, K. Juhila, M. Matarese and C. van Nijnatten (eds) *Analysing Social Work Communication: Discourse in practice* (pp. 98–116), London: Routledge.

Hall, C., Slembrouck, S. and Sarangi, S. (2006) *Language Practices in Social Work: Categorisation and accountability in child welfare*, London: Routledge.

Hall, C., Slembrouck, S., Haig, E. and Lee, A. (2010) "The management of professional and other roles during boundary work in child welfare", *International Journal of Social Welfare*, 19(3): 348–357.

Harris, J., Borodkina, O., Brodtkorb, E., Evans, T., Kessl, F., Schnurr, S. and Slettebo, T. (2015) "International travelling knowledge in social work: an analytic framework", *European Journal of Social Work*, 18(4): 481–494.

Heritage, J. (1984) *Garfinkel and Ethnomethodology*, Cambridge: Polity.

Heritage, J. (2001) "Goffman, Garfinkel and conversation analysis", in M. Wetherell, S. Taylor and S.J. Yates (eds) *Discourse Theory and Practice: A reader* (pp. 47–56), London: Sage.

Heritage, J. and Atkinson, J.M. (1984) "Introduction", in J.M. Atkinson and J. Heritage (eds) *Structures of Social Action: Studies in conversation analysis* (pp. 1–15), Cambridge: Cambridge University Press.

Heritage, J. and Sefi, S. (1992) "Dilemmas of advice: aspects of the delivery and reception of advice in interactions between health visitors and first time mothers", in P. Drew and J. Heritage (eds) *Talk at work: Interaction in institutional settings* (pp. 359–417), Cambridge: Cambridge University Press.

Hernes, T. (2004) "Studying composite boundaries: a framework of analysis", *Human Relations*, 57(1): 9–29.

Hester, S. and Eglin, P. (eds) (1997a) *Culture in Action: Studies in membership categorization analysis*, Lanham, MD: International Institute for Ethnomethodology and University Press of America.

Hester, S. and Eglin, P. (1997b) "Membership categorization analysis: an introduction", in S. Hester and P. Eglin (eds) *Culture in Action: Studies in membership categorization analysis* (pp. 1–23), Lanham; MD: International Institute for Ethnomethodology and Conversation Analysis and University Press of America.

Hindmarsh, N. and Llewellyn, J. (2010) "Finding organization in detail: methodological orientations", in J. Llewellyn and N. Hindmarsh (eds) *Organisation, Interaction and Practice: Studies in ethnomethodology and conversation analysis* (pp. 24–45), Cambridge: Cambridge University Press.

Hjörne, E., Juhila, K. and van Nijnatten, C. (2010) "Negotiating dilemmas in the practices of street-level welfare work", *International Journal of Social Welfare*, 19(3): 303–309.

Jameson, F. (1981) *The Political Unconscious: Narrative as a socially symbolic act*, London: Methuen.

Jayyusi, L. (1991) "Values and moral judgement: communicative praxis as a moral order", in G. Button (ed.) *Ethnomethodology and the Human Sciences* (pp. 227–251), Cambridge: Cambridge University Press.

Jefferson, G. and Lee, J. (1992) "The rejection of advice: managing the problematic convergence of a 'troubles-telling' and a 'service encounter'", in P. Drew and J. Heritage (eds) *Talk at Work: Interaction in institutional settings* (pp. 521–548), Cambridge: Cambridge University Press.

Juhila, K. (2004) "Talking back to stigmatised identities: negotiation of culturally dominant categorizations in interviews with shelter residents", *Qualitative Social Work*, 3(3): 259–275.

Juhila, K., Caswell, D. and Raitakari, S. (2014a) "Resistance", in C. Hall, K. Juhila, M. Matarese and C. van Nijnatten (eds) *Analysing Social Work Communication: Discourse in practice* (pp. 117–135), London: Routledge.

Juhila, K., Hall, C. and Raitakari, S. (2010) "Accounting for the clients' troublesome behaviour in a supported housing unit: blames, excuses and responsibility in professionals' talk", *Journal of Social Work*, 10(1): 59–79.

Juhila, K., Mäkitalo, Å. and Noordegraaf, N. (2014b) "Analysing social work interaction: premises and approaches", in C. Hall, K. Juhila, M. Matarese and C. van Nijnatten (eds) *Analysing Social Work Communication: Discourse in practice* (pp. 9–24), London: Routledge.

Koskiaho, B. (2008) *Hyvinvointipalvelujen tavaratalossa* [In the department store of welfare services], Tampere: Vastapaino.

Labov, W. (1972) *Language in the Inner City: Studies in the black English vernacular*, Pittsburgh: University of Pennsylvania Press.

Lamont, M. and Molnár, V. (2002) "The study of boundaries in the social sciences", *Annual Review of Sociology*, 28(1): 167–195.

Lipsky, M. (1980) *Street-level Bureaucracy: Dilemmas of the individual in public services*, New York: Russell Sage Foundation.

Llewellyn, J. and Hindmarsh, N. (2010) "Work and organization in real time: an introduction", in J. Llewellyn and N. Hindmarsh (eds) *Organisation, Interaction and Practice: Studies in ethnomethodology and conversation analysis* (pp. 3–23), Cambridge: Cambridge University Press.

MacMartin, C. (2008) "Resisting optimistic questions in narrative and solution-focused therapies", in A. Peräkylä, C. Antaki, S. Vehviläinen and I. Leudar (eds) *Conversation Analysis and Psychotherapy* (pp. 80–99), Cambridge: Cambridge University Press.

Martin, D. (2007) "Responsibility: a philosophical perspective", in G. Dewsbury and J. Dobson (eds) *Responsibility and Dependable System* (pp. 21–42), London: Springer.

Matarese, M. and Caswell, D. (2014) "Accountability", in C. Hall, K. Juhila, M. Matarese and C. Van Nijnatten (eds) *Analysing Social Work Communication: Discourse in practice* (pp. 44–60), London: Routledge.

Maynard, D.W. (1988) "Language, interaction and social problems", *Social Problems*, 35(4): 311–334.

Miller, P. and Rose, N. (2008) *Governing the Present: Administering economic, social and personal life*, Cambridge: Polity Press.

Morley, D. and Silverstone, R. (1990) "Domestic communication: technologies and meanings", *Media, Culture & Society*, 12(1): 31–55.

Mäkitalo, Å. (2003) "Accounting practices and situated knowing: dilemmas and dynamics in institutional categorization", *Discourse Studies*, 5(4): 495–516.

Mäkitalo, Å. (2014) "Categorisation", in C. Hall, K. Juhila, M. Matarese and C. van Nijnatten (eds) *Analysing Social Work Communication: Discourse in practice* (pp. 25–43), London: Routledge.

Ochs, E. and Capps, L. (2001) *Living Narrative: Creating lives in everyday storytelling*, Cambridge, MA: Harvard University Press.

Osvaldsson, K. (2004). " 'I don't have no damn cultures': doing normality in a 'deviant' setting", *Qualitative Research in Psychology*, 1(3): 239–264.

Pomerantz, A. (1978) "Attributions of responsibility: blamings", *Sociology*, 12(1): 115–121.

Potter, J. (2002) "Two kinds of natural", *Discursive Studies*, 4(2): 539–542.

Potter, J. and Hepburn, A. (2010) "A kind of governance: rules, time and psychology in organizations", in J. Llewellyn and N. Hindmarsh (eds) *Organisation, Interaction and Practice: Studies in ethnomethodology and conversation analysis* (pp. 49–73), Cambridge: Cambridge University Press.

Prottas, J.M. (1979) *People-processing: The street-level bureaucrat in public service bureaucracies*, Toronto: Lexington Books.

Psathas, G. (1995) *Conversation Analysis: The study of talk-in-interaction*, London: Sage, Qualitative Research Methods Series 35.

Riessman, C. (2008) *Narrative Methods for the Human Sciences*, London: Sage.

Riessman, C. and Quinney, L. (2005) "Narrative in social work: a critical review", *Qualitative Social Work*, 4(4): 391–412.

Rosulek, L. (2010) "Legitimation and the heteroglossic nature of closing arguments", in D. Schiffrin, A. De Fina and A. Nylund (eds) *Telling stories: Language, narrative and social life* (pp. 181–194), Washington, DC: Georgetown University Press.

Saario, S., Juhila, K. and Raitakari, S. (2015) "Boundary work in inter-agency and inter-professional client transitions", *Interprofessional Journal of Care*, 29(6): 610–615.

Sacks, H. (1972a) "An initial investigation of the usability of conversational data for doing sociology", in D. Sudnow (ed.) *Studies in Social Interaction* (pp. 31–74), New York: Free Press.

Sacks, H. (1972b) "On the analyzability of stories by children", In J. Coulter (ed.) *Ethnomethodological Sociology* (pp. 254–270), Aldershot, UK: Edward Elgar Publishing Company.

Sacks, H. (1992). *Lectures on Conversation*, Volume I. Oxford: Blackwell.

Sacks, H., Schegloff, E. and Jefferson, G. (1974) "A simplest systematics for the organization of turn-taking for conversation", *Language*, 50(4): 696–735.

Schatzki, T.R. (2001) "Introduction: practice theory", in T.R. Schatzki, K. Knorr Cetina and E. von Savigny (eds) *The Practice Turn in Contemporary Theory* (pp. 1–14), London: Routledge.

Schatzki, T.R., Knorr Cetina, K. and von Savigny, E. (eds) (2001) *The Practice Turn in Contemporary Theory*, London: Routledge.

Scott, M. and Lyman, S. (1968) "Accounts", *American Sociological Review*, 33(1): 46–62.

Silverman, D. (1997) *Discourses of Counselling: HIV counselling as social interaction.* London: Sage.

Silverman, D. (2007) *A Very Short, Fairly Interesting and Reasonably Cheap Book about Qualitative Research*, London: Sage.

Slembrouck, S. and Hall, C. (2014) "Boundary work", in C. Hall, K. Juhila, M. Matarese and C. van Nijnatten (eds) *Analysing Social Work Communication: Discourse in practice* (pp. 61–78), London: Routledge.

Solberg, J. (2011) "Accepted and resisted: the client's responsibility for making proposals in activation encounters", *Text & Talk*, 31(6): 733–752.

Vehviläinen, S. (1999) *Structures of Counselling Interaction: A conversation analytic study of counselling encounters in career guidance training*, Helsinki: Helsinki University Press.

Virokannas, E. (2011) "Identity categorization of motherhood in the context of drug abuse and child welfare services, *Qualitative Social Work*, 10(3): 329–345.

Wikström, E. (2008) "Boundary work as inner and outer dialogue: dieticians in Sweden", *Qualitative Research in Organizations and Management: An International Journal*, 3(1): 59–77.

Zimmerman, D.H. (1998) "Identity, context and interaction", in C. Antaki and S. Widdicombe (eds) *Identities in Talk* (pp. 87–106), London: Sage.

Part II
Managing client responsibilities

5 Clients accounting for the responsible self in interviews

Suvi Raitakari and Kirsi Günther

Introduction

Nowadays, lively political and academic discussions revolve around the issue of personal and social responsibilities (e.g. Passini 2011; Snelling 2012; Pearl and Lebowitz 2014). For example, the discussions consider in what sense and to what extent (ill)-health and (bad) well-being are personal choices and accomplishments (Giddens 1999; Wikler 2002; Brownell *et al.* 2010; Scott and Wilson 2011; Wiley *et al.* 2013). A common view is that individuals are primarily responsible for their health and well-being and thus at least partly causing their adversities and problems (Robert *et al.* 2008; Lundell *et al.* 2013). Although public perceptions are not monolithic and this view of the responsible self is widely criticised, it can still be said to represent a dominant cultural expectation of agency in the Western world (Lyon-Callo 2000; Pearl and Lebowitz 2014).

Clients who use employment, health, social and housing services and benefits are culturally expected to account for being responsible and "trying", despite their need for subsidies and support services. However, individuals experiencing social exclusion are often in a difficult position due to attempting to live up to the idea of a responsible self. Social exclusion erases and narrows capabilities, resources and choices in life, and can be defined as "what can happen when people or areas suffer from a combination of linked problems such as unemployment, poor skills, low incomes, unfair discrimination, poor housing, high crime, bad health, and family breakdown" (Social Exclusion Unit 2004: 4; Cole *et al.* 2011: 13). These features are also well-known social determinations of (mental) health problems (SDH) (Lundell *et al.* 2013: 1116; May *et al.* 2013).

One root of the responsibility discussion is advanced liberalism that emphasises that people are to help themselves and find ways to strengthen their capabilities to be self-governing individuals. Personal responsibility and self-management are widely discussed in the governmentality literature (Rose 1996; Scott and Wilson 2011; Solberg 2011; Chapter 2 of this volume). Interestingly, self-management, which implies empowerment and recovery, is at present strongly promoted in the (margins of) welfare services (Davidson 2005; Scott and Wilson 2011; Chapter 3 of this volume). For instance, self-management has become a common approach in mental health work (Sterling *et al.* 2010), as illustrated in the client interview data examples in this chapter. Often, welfare workers support the client's responsibility and ability to manage his/her difficulties in life by conducting self-management techniques, such as making weekly programmes and schedules with the clients. Self-management can be understood as the ability of individuals to get along with the symptoms as well as the physical, psychosocial and lifestyle changes inherent in living with severe conditions (e.g. by learning to utilise different techniques and welfare services) (Johnston *et al.* 2008). Thus, it first and foremost puts forward the notion of personal responsibility in line with advanced liberalism.

Our aim in this chapter is to reflect on issues related to personal and social responsibilities by applying the concept of self-management, which we understand as being a mediator between macro-level discussions on responsibilities, professionals' ideas of good recovery and grass-roots level practices at the margins of welfare services. The question addressed is as follows: how do clients manage personal and social responsibilities in the process of recovery at the time of rising expectations of self-management and the responsible self (self-responsibilisation)?

We begin by introducing discussions related to responsibility and self-management. Discourses of responsibility can roughly be divided into two: those that emphasise personal responsibility as essential in one's agency and well-being (Brownell *et al.* 2010), and those that concentrate on social responsibility i.e. that emphasise that other people, institutions and collectives are crucial for ensuring an individual's well-being in society. Personal responsibility can especially be seen as a crucial element of becoming the subject of one's life (see Giddens 1999; McNamee and Gergen 1999; Kelty 2008; Ballet *et al.* 2007), whilst social responsibility emphasises the subjects' interconnected relations and obligations: "the importance of connections between people, through their social commitments and their embedding in social institutions" (Ballet *et al.* 2007: 186). Accordingly, personal and social responsibility intersect with one another, as a responsible self is not only expected to manage one's own life but also to be socially enlightened and to take care of the well-being of others (Rose 1996; Lister 2015).

We then continue by demonstrating via interview data examples how, on the one hand, clients at the margins of welfare services account for taking (or trying to take) responsibility for themselves and others, and, on the other hand, they resist this cultural expectation as impossible to live up to (in a current situation). There exists a gap between cultural expectations and the resources and capabilities of individuals (Scott and Lyman 1968). This gap is present in the interview talk, in the form of excuses, justifications and explanations in regard to expectations of restoring things back to "normal" in a responsible way (see Chapter 4). In the analysis section, we illustrate how clients reflect on the discourses of responsibility and self-management. These discourses set norms for good and respected individuals, and thus they offer "yardsticks" for the clients to assess their self-management abilities and stages of recovery.

Discourses constructing the responsible self

Discourses of responsibility

> As it is used today, "responsibility" is an interestingly ambiguous or multi-layered term. In one sense, someone who is responsible for an event can be said to be the author of that event. This is the original sense of "respons-ible", which links it with causality or agency. Another meaning of respons-ibility is where we speak of someone being responsible if he or she acts in an ethical or accountable manner. Responsibility also however means obligation, or liability, and this is the most interesting sense to counterpose with risk.
>
> (Giddens 1999: 8)

In line with the above quotation, Snelling's (2012: 162) definition demonstrates the multi-faced nature of responsibility. He represents a three-dimensional defi-nition of responsibility: "(i) a responsible agent; (ii) having obligations (respons-ibilities); and (iii) being susceptible to being held responsible (that is blamed if he fails to meet them)". Responsibilities can, as in this chapter, be approached as discursive accomplishments that are constantly redefined and revised in par-ticular contexts and social situations. This is what we mean by the term "dis-courses of responsibility".

Responsibilities are expressed in relation to authorities and governance, and thus they imply existing power relations, obligations and rules related to pre-ferred behaviour and actions in present-day society. Individuals have rights and responsibilities with respect to each other, communities, social institutions and authorities (Dean 2002; Flynn 2005; Ballet *et al.* 2007; Kelty 2008; Passini 2011: 282). As Trnka and Trundle (2014: 136) argue, "responsibility is a multi-valent concept and practice that is central to contemporary social life. Notions of responsibility are pervasive, visible in forms of governance, emerging and endur-ing subjectivities, and collective relations in a wide range of settings." For example, being a welfare client implies particular responsibilities set by the welfare professionals and institutions. Also, the status of being a human being in Western society distributes responsibilities and rights to individuals according to human rights, religion and democracy. All in all, discourses of responsibility govern and direct individual conduct. However, they comprise a dispersed and conflicting totality that makes it possible for the individual to act upon the idea of the responsible self in various ways in different personal, societal and interac-tional contexts. Discourses of responsibility therefore enable and prompt agency in many ways, yet also restrict it.

Doheny (2007) deals with discourses of responsibility by presenting a liberal, republican, communitarian and deliberative democratic version of responsibility. Liberal responsibility is mostly about personal rights and responsibilities. It emphasises the importance of not abusing or misusing the rights of a free individual, whereas republican and communitarian versions have more to say about social responsibilities as civic virtues (see also Lister 2015). From a critical point of view, it can be argued that although republican and communitarian versions of responsibility "explain that the citizen must internalize certain virtues if s/he is to behave responsibly, there is an absence of detail on how the responsible citizen grapples with their actual responsibilities" (Doheny 2007: 408). The deliberative democratic version of responsibility, which is introduced as an alternative and preferred version of responsibility, highlights that a fair distribution of responsibilities requires ethical sensitiveness, reflective thinking and negotiations. It is also seen to offer a relevant theoretical background to understand how people tackle responsibility issues in their everyday life. Following the idea of responsibilities being negotiated and managed at the grass-roots level, it has been studied, for example, how patient responsibility is constructed and negotiated in hospital settings and "how these practices draw on discourses of medicine, care and neo-liberalism" (Holen and Ahrenkiel 2011: 299). Similarly Beckmann (2013) studies lived experiences of people living with HIV/AIDS in Tanzania, and how they account for acting responsibly according to their condition, even though the biomedical authorities often see this action as irresponsible.

As discussed in this book, Miller and Rose (e.g. 2008) have approached personal responsibility as a representation of an advanced liberal form of governance that is known for relying on and enabling individual independence, empowerment and self-management (Rose 1996; Dean 2002; Chapter 2 of this volume). In other words, advanced liberal governance values self-disciplined, multi-skilled, entrepreneurial and resilient individuals (Stasiulis and Bakan 2003: 22; Ilcan 2009: 211; Solberg 2011). As Hazleden (2014: 422) sees it: "Contemporary understandings and classification of the self are bound up with (neo) liberal political ideology and the rhetoric of choice, self-responsibility and individual aspiration". The advanced liberal understanding of personal responsibility is often referred to as "self-responsibilisation". This stresses personal choice and autonomy as the means through which personal responsibility is accomplished – the state's responsibilities are reduced, and it is up to the individual to make the best out of the opportunities and to reach for the best possible well-being. As Michailakis and Schirmer (2010: 931) put it, we have witnessed a "shift from a collective responsibility of the welfare state towards individual responsibility". Self-responsibilisation focuses on how clients' personal subjectivities are shaped by advanced liberal political expectations (Hazleden 2014: 433). Accordingly, individual agency is directed by ongoing (self-)responsibilisation accounting processes (Clarke 2005).

Client responsibility and self-management

Personal responsibility is strongly addressed in client responsibility and self-management approaches. Holding individuals accountable for their lifestyle choices and health is both a general and topical, yet controversial, discussion in today's society, which has a growing awareness of health risks, the importance of prevention and the growing demands for more and better treatments for lower costs (Cappelen and Norheim 2005; Cayton 2006; Jallinoja *et al.* 2007; Share and Strain 2008; Civaner and Arda 2008: 267; Michailakis and Schirmer 2010; Scott and Wilson 2011). Civaner and Arda (2008: 264) have come up with the following list of patient responsibilities:

> promoting self-health, respect for the health and well-being of others, the appropriate use of health care resources in the public sector, sharing relevant health information with health care workers, considering carefully any advice offered by the health care worker, and adhering to agreed treatment plans.

They classify patient responsibilities into four categories: "technical requirements, consumer obligations, responsibility for one's own health, and responsibilities to society at large (social responsibility)" (Civaner and Arda 2008: 264). Holen and Ahrenkiel's (2011) study shows that patient responsibility comprises aspects such as having morality, possessing proper will, being compliant, displaying control and controllability, being active and, most importantly, striving for self-sufficiency.

Self-management resonates with, and has been incorporated into, patient/client responsibility discussions (Jallinoja *et al.* 2007: 244), and it was first applied in the welfare work context in the medical rehabilitation and chronic disease literature (Sterling *et al.* 2010: 133). The approach is based on and promotes the idea of a health consumer who is a responsible, choosing, life-planning and self-efficient actor (Scott and Wilson 2011: 43). Within this approach, the ideal client is one who monitors and governs his/her condition with the help of appropriate expert knowledge and support. It expects the client to perform responsibly also by pursuing healthy living and reducing risks, following chosen care plans and medication, and being a co-operative and active actor in the health and social services (Lorig and Holman 2003; Sterling *et al.* 2010: 134). The expertise of welfare workers is directed particularly to "individuals who lack the cognitive, emotional, practical and ethical skills to take the personal responsibility for rational self-management" (Rose 1996: 348).

In the governmentality literature, self-management programmes are named as "responsibility projects" (see Chapter 2). Self-management can be interpreted to focus on "inquiring about the self", which is also a bedrock of advanced liberalism governance, as the majority of its techniques for tackling social problems "fall under the rubric of self-help and governing of the self" (Lyon-Callo 2000: 335; see also Broom *et al.* 2014). Rose (1990) calls techniques that focus on the transformation of subjectivity from powerlessness to active participation as "technologies of citizenship" (Hazleden 2014: 423; see Chapter 6 of this volume). Accordingly, the self-management approach is said to be "social revolution, not against capitalism, racism, and gender inequality, but against the order of the self and the way we govern ourselves" (Cruikshank 1996: 231 ref. Lyon-Callo 2000: 335).

In addition, the self-management approach implies empowerment and recovery (Davidson 2005; Johnston *et al.* 2008; Sterling *et al.* 2010; Pulvirenti *et al.* 2014; Chapter 3 of this volume). It is enhanced by stating that when clients are actively involved in managing their conditions, better outcomes are achieved. It is also seen as the client's right to have an active role in finding solutions to health and well-being problems. In other words, self-management permits clients to become participants in the recovery process (Davidson 2005; Sterling *et al.* 2010; Chapter 3 of this volume). The approach is applied as a professional care ideology, as programmes and specific techniques to strengthen and empower clients to overcome difficulties and improve their quality of life despite possible lifelong conditions. In long-term conditions, self-management is seen as a life-long learning process and task that can be accomplished and strengthened by mutual co-operation between clients and welfare workers. Johnston *et al.* (2008: 5) state that "at the heart of each self-management approach is an empowered patient with the skills and confidence to better manage chronic diseases and interact with the primary health care system". They also provide an enlightening definition of self-management that emphasises empowerment and reciprocal relationship between clients and welfare workers:

> Self-management refers to an individual's ability to manage the symptoms, treatment, physical, psychosocial, and lifestyle changes inherent in living with a chronic condition. Self-management programmes seek to empower individuals to cope with disease and live better quality lives with fewer restrictions from their illness by developing self-efficacy, which is the level of confidence that an individual has in his or her ability to succeed in dealing with their own chronic disease. It is important to note the distinction between initiatives to build patient self-management and self-management support. Self-management support requires a provider or health care team to perform a certain set of tasks to create the self-efficacy necessary for a patient to deal confidently with their own range of emotional, physical, and physiological symptoms of their chronic disease. Self-management does not replace a health care team, but rather, encourages a reciprocal relationship between patient and physician, where self-management skills can be built and used at home, as well as in routine health care system interactions.
>
> (Johnston *et al.* 2008: 5)

This definition links together personal and social responsibility, as workers are constructed as the ones enabling, via reciprocal relationship, a client to be self-efficient in the community. To grasp how clients manage severe conditions in everyday contexts, it is important to understand their ways of making sense of everyday challenges, health, ill-health and their agency; and the structural barriers that hinder their access to resources. Clients often are in a position where they have no other alternatives than to balance the demands of the condition against those of everyday life, and to manage in one way or another with or without the support of welfare workers (see van Houtum *et al.* 2015). Clients thus display personal responsibility, agency and means to manage difficulties and risks, even though their actions might not always be approved by welfare workers. The self-management approach is based on three presumptions that need to be addressed cautiously. First, individuals are seen as disempowered per se. Second, it is assumed that all individuals want or have the resources to be empowered, to make life changes or to self-manage their conditions in a professionally preferred way (Pulvirenti *et al.* 2014). Third, it is an individual client that is worked on and targeted for interventions. A critical stance towards the self-management approach and its presumptions makes it possible to resist the cultural expectation of the responsible self and to recognise its limits and risks, such as victim blaming (see Chapter 2) – without denying the positive consequences of the approach for clients' agency and well-being.

Clients taking part in life management programmes and techniques

Self-management programmes and specific techniques are at present commonly conducted in welfare services to enhance the self-efficacy and personal skills of clients to govern health and welfare difficulties in everyday settings (Lorig *et al.* 1994; Lorig and Holman 2003; Sterling *et al.* 2010; Cramm *et al.* 2015). It can be argued that the self-management approach currently represents a preferred way to do mental health work and to understand client participation. In the following, we briefly introduce a few self-management programmes to demonstrate how they construct the client as a responsible and active participant in service delivery and thus promote the cultural expectation of the responsible self.

Different self-management programmes – for instance, Care Programme Approach (CPA) (see Chapter 7), Wellness Recovery Action Planning (WRAP) and Recovery Star – comprise techniques such as education, care plans, timetables, advice-giving and directing, agreements, self-assessments and follow-ups to achieve recovery and better ability to function. WRAP is one of the mental health self-management techniques developed by service users and rooted in the recovery movement. It is widely applied, especially in English-speaking countries (Davidson 2005; Doughty *et al.* 2008; Scott and Wilson 2011). Scott and Wilson (2011: 40) take a critical stance towards it and note: "The WRAP is noteworthy for its construction of a health identity which is individualised, responsibilised, and grounded in an 'at risk' subjectivity; success with this programme requires development of an intensely focused health lifestyle".

Recovery Star is a holistic and personalised outcome measurement tool. It is based on the idea that both the worker and the client assess, rate and discuss the client's progress in self-management and recovery. The tool directs clients to plan, quantify and reflect on their progress, and welfare professionals and organisations to capture performance and outcome results (Onifade 2011; Tickle *et al.* 2013). Ten dimensions (see Dickens *et al.* 2012) are assessed: "managing mental health; physical health and self-care, living skills, social networks, work, relationships, addictive behavior, responsibilities, identity and self-esteem and trust and hope" (Tickle *et al.* 2013: 195). Furthermore, Recovery Star is based on the idea of a "ladder of change" that demonstrates steps in the recovery journey from "being stuck to accepting help, then on to believing that things can change, thereafter to learning new skills/approaches to maintain recovery and finally to self-reliance" (Onifade 2011). Like WRAP, Recovery Star aims to construct and facilitate transformation from a passive self driven by external forces to a reflexive self that is proactively and responsibly managing the circumstances and difficulties in life.

The clients, whose interview talk we analyse in this chapter, have participated in a range of self-management programmes with varying degrees of strictness. They have been clients of several health and social services, having lived in supported housing and rehabilitation course settings, or independently with the support of floating support services. Accordingly, our presumption is that they have confronted and experienced a range of "re-responsibilisation" techniques, such as monitoring pre-symptoms and well-being, making weekly schedules, taking part in self-care groups, practising social and everyday living skills, and receiving advice concerning healthy living, medication and preferred behaviour. Thus, it is important to scrutinise how such "re-responsibilised", and in many ways socially excluded, individuals account for personal and social responsibility.

Clients accounting for causes and responsibilities in interview talk

> To live a life at all is to confront conditions that are nettlesome, disappointing, irritating, and downright devastating. The problem then is not that we confront the problematic but, rather, how we respond. Perhaps the chief riposte is to seek restoration: We strive to ascertain cause and with cause in place, gain rationale for action. With responsibility assigned, we sense responsibilities for admonishment, correction, coercion, punishment, and so on.
>
> (McNamee and Gergen 1999: 3)

Responsibility is a central concept within human life and thus also for an ethnomethodologically informed research approach (see Chapter 4) where it is seen as linked to accountability in social interaction. Following this approach, the subsequent analysis examines negotiations of responsibilities "in action". We ask: to what extent and in what ways do the clients (and interviewers) orient to the discourses of responsibility and self-management approach in interview interaction?

The illustrative examples are chosen from a data corpus of 44 (32 Finnish and 12 English) client interviews, which have been conducted in four different settings:

1   a supported housing and floating support service for people with mental health and substance abuse problems (Finland);
2   a floating support service for people with mental health problems (UK);

3   a project offering housing and social skills training for young adults with diagnosed schizophrenia (Finland);
4   an outpatient clinic for people with severe drug abuse problems (Finland).

All these services are run by non-governmental organisations (NGOs) (see Chapter 4). The services deploy a variety of self-management programmes and techniques to promote individual recovery and coping in everyday life. For example, the clients commonly practice travelling by public transport, and everyday living skills such as cooking and cleaning. An essential activity is also giving information about mental difficulties and substance abuse problems and advising how to manage them.

The structure of the thematic interview was the same in England and Finland. The interview proceeded temporally: the themes addressed the past, present and future hopes of clients. The themes covered the clients' background, previous and present accommodation, and contacts with the social and health services. In addition, direct questions were asked about agency, personal and social responsibility, and client-centredness.

Responsibilities are often touched upon by both participants in the interviews: by the interviewer when putting forward questions in a frame of responsibility and self-management, and thus inviting the client to give an account of their own responsibilities and those of others. As seen from the examples, the interviewer directs interviews by asking questions that imply particular presumptions concerning the client roles and responsibilities in the recovery process. However, the main emphasis in the analysis is on the responses and accounting practices of clients (not on the expressions of the interviewers).

In the analysis, we apply analytical concepts such as causal accounting and resistance (see Chapter 4). In a broad sense, accounts are seen to be present in all everyday communication (e.g. Buttny 1993; Antaki 1994). In accounting, speakers address issues of agency and responsibility (Edwards and Potter 1993: 25). As Garfinkel (1967: 33) notes, speakers routinely build into their talk accounts rebuttals to potential criticisms (see Raitakari *et al.* 2013). For example, in interview talk clients often explain their action and answer questions in a way that implies that they are aware that they are potentially judged as "not responsible" and "not trying". As Matarese and Caswell (2014: 46) state, "accounts are common responses to questions prompting an explanation".

When we apply a narrower sub-concept of accounting – causal accounting – the interest lies in how individuals account for causes and construct cause-and-effect relations when making sense of their actions and the situation at hand (Bull and Shaw 1992; Juhila *et al.* 2010). By "cause-and-effect relation", we do not refer to mechanistic causality, as in experimental methods, but to individuals' everyday rhetorical claims of cause-and-effect (Bull and Shaw 1992; Raitakari *et al.* 2013). Applying Bull and Shaw's (1992) ideas on causal accounting, we scrutinise the clients' "theories of cause" and how they construct relations between causes, agency and responsibilities regarding their own situations and behaviour. In a variety of ways, the clients claim causal relations between the following issues:

What is causing their conditions and difficulties? What can be done to ease the suffering? Who ought to be active and responsible in solving problems?

By giving causes, justifications and explanations – for example, by referring to factors that are out of one's reach or control, or are unchangeable – individuals define the scope of their responsibilities and account for not being able to be the expected responsible self. In the client interview talk, causal accounts are often built in a manner that creates an image of a good client who is trying his/her best in a demanding situation to live according to self-management expectations. However, the clients also construct causal accounts that imply resistance towards and resigning from the self-management approach.

The analysis section proceeds in the following way. In the first part, we analyse data examples that illustrate accounts of trying to be the responsible self. We notice that the clients often express their wish to be more self-sufficient, independent and active in life, but at the same time there are things that make it impossible for them. We refer to this kind of talk when using the term "trying to be the responsible self". We chose, named and organised the data examples according to different factors that the clients construct as being mainly their responsibility. In the second part, we examine data examples that illustrate resistance towards personal responsibility. This resisting talk produces causal accounts for not being able to be responsible for one's life (for now) or act responsibly (in a particular situation). It also makes it possible for the client to question the profound justification of (re)-responsibilisation. Accordingly, we have named the last data examples according to the reasons constructed as explanations and justifications of why the client is not capable of taking the position of the responsible self. Hence, the analysis in a general sense demonstrates how discourses of responsibility and self-management are reflected among clients at the margins of welfare services.

Responsible self: accounting for trying

Responsible for ...

Our first impression of the data was that it comprises a large amount of professional self-management vocabularies, as well as causal accounts that explain why it is difficult for the clients to live up to the expectation of the responsible self as much as they would like to. These causal accounts also imply attributes of responsibility and blame. The clients describe their struggles with ordinary everyday matters and limited resources, yet also their abilities to manage symptoms and to estimate their shifting ability to function. Whilst doing this, they simultaneously allocate responsibilities to themselves and others – for example, welfare workers.

... managing care contacts, monitoring oneself and seeking help

The first example is client interview data from England. The client is living in her own flat with the support of a floating support service. She is in her fifties and has special needs related to substance abuse and severe psychotic-level mental health problems. The interview is held in a supported housing and floating support service's office. The data excerpt is from an interview section concerning support services and professional networks taking part in the client's treatment.

Extract 1

1 INTERVIEWER: What is important for your own well-being?
2 CLIENT: Making sure that I'm drug-free and alcohol-free, that's the most important one. Making sure that I have three teams, Support Service, my advocate and my psychiatrist and my social worker. Making sure they're there so I can trust them. So that if I do start to feel unwell, I have somebody that I can phone up, you know, and get in touch with. Instead of leaving it and leaving it, and getting worse, you know, to the point where I want to hurt myself. I don't want to have to get to that point any more.

At the beginning of the extract, the interviewer asks what is important for the client in sustaining her well-being (turn 1). In the response the client constructs herself as being personally responsible for "*making sure that I'm drug-free and alcohol-free*". Her duty is "*making sure*" about a variety of things: a substance-free life, support services, a trustworthy worker and her ability to act if things are "*getting worse, you know, to the point where I want to hurt myself*". In her response, the client portrays herself as a strong and empowered agent in the sense that she manages her condition and professional network, monitors well-being, makes requests for support and allocates appropriate responsibility to the welfare workers. Causal accounts are presented when the client argues that she is required to be active in order to sustain good condition and support relations. Conversely, she constructs her possible passivity as a cause that leads to a worsening of things. The client wants to be the responsible self who takes care and does not hurt herself. However, success in this is bound to her ability to be proactive and keeping the welfare workers committed to helping her. In her response, the client displays herself as an active actor who is responsible for arranging her own care. She positions herself as the central person whose role is to inform, co-ordinate and make demands on welfare workers concerning her health and safety. The responsibility to manage the condition is constructed as being shared between the client and welfare workers; responsibilities are based on reciprocal client–worker relationships. In order for the client to act responsibly, the welfare workers carry an obligation to be available and responsive to the client's needs.

In general, such client talk reflects the ideals of the personal responsibility and self-management approach. The self is constructed as being active, reflexive, monitoring and responsible for the condition getting better or worse. Accordingly, the client associates with personal responsibility and self-management vocabularies, and this makes it possible for her to display strong and empowered agency. However, the client's ability to be personally responsible is bound to the welfare workers' social responsibility to be liable and available to care for the client.

... being an independent and well-functioning client

The following data example is from a client interview conducted in the Finnish project offering housing and social skills training for young adults with diagnosed schizophrenia. The client is in his thirties and has a severe mental health problem, which makes coping in everyday life demanding. The interview is held in the project's office. The excerpt is from the end of the interview, where the client's wishes for the future are being discussed.

Extract 2

1   INTERVIEWER: Well. You can choose yourself. Thinking about something so extensive as the future. What would you ...

2   CLIENT: Hope for?

3   INTERVIEWER: Hope for?

4   CLIENT: Well. Functional capacity, to be able to do those things that I used to do, which I was interested in. Difficult.

5   INTERVIEWER: Functional capacity is fairly broad too and it comprises so many issues.

6   CLIENT: Yeah, and I also want this, what would I call it? It's a bit difficult to describe. Functional capacity and what else? This kind of, like having a tolerable life somehow. So I wouldn't have to suffer so damn much. That kind of thing.

7   INTERVIEWER: Well, that's something already.

8   CLIENT: Well, anyway, functional capacity and coping in life. I could get started with that. And managing symptoms. I mean, they're mostly the same things as here [project's name].

9   INTERVIEWER: Indeed. Yeah, you do have plenty to hope for there.

10 CLIENT: To be able to finally become independent despite everything. Not be so dependent on so many things just because you're so broken.

11 INTERVIEWER: Do you think that becoming independent would be about having less contact with these treatment places, or ...

12 CLIENT: I mean just in general, to have enough money, the apartment would be in decent shape, financial issues would be handled on time and accurately without any changes to payment terms or due dates, and things like that. It also requires that I should get this chaos out of my head somehow.

The extract begins with the interviewer's inquiry concerning the client's future expectations (turn 1). The client first clarifies that the question is really about his wishes (turn 2). Then he responds by using professional self-management language: "*functional capacity and coping in life. I could get started with that. And managing symptoms. I mean, they're mostly the same things as here [project's name]*" (turn 8). In this turn, the client explicitly makes a reference to the project that is underway that can be regarded as a specific self-management programme. The client hopes for the same things that have been discussed in the project. He uses causal accounting when arguing that the limited ability to function is restricting him from doing things that he has previously done and that would interest him (turn 4). Poor ability to function is thus constructed as a cause and a justification of a passive self.

The client continues by constructing himself as trying to be eventually more independent and less dependent "*despite everything*" (turn 10). The client justifies his current dependency by defining himself as incomplete: "*you're so broken*". An "incomplete" self cannot be independent and thus is constructed as the cause of the client being dependent. The client expresses dependency negatively: he values independence, and wants to abandon dependency although he has restrictions. Independence is culturally a highly appreciated attribute of the responsible self, and it is for the client, too. The interviewer presents a clarifying question concerning what independency actually means for the client, and suggests that it might mean having less intense relations with the treatment institutions (in this way aligning with the idea of independence being a valued attribute, turn 11).

However, the client talks into being a more overall self-management-based understanding of independence. He stresses the following issues: "*to have enough money, the apartment would be in decent shape, financial issues would be handled on time and accurately without any changes to payment terms or due dates, and things like that*". These resonate with the expectations related to the responsible self (turn 12). The client thus recognises improved self-management as his future recovery aim, yet also constructs a major obstacle to achieving it: "*It also requires that I should get this chaos out of my head somehow*". The client uses the passive tense. Hence, from the utterance, it is possible to read what the client is displaying as his aim and what the difficulty is in reaching it, but it is not possible to read who would be able to undo the difficulty, and how; the chaos. The utterance is constructed as a causal account: the mental chaos is seen as causing the dependency, and consequently to achieve independence, the chaos first needs to be solved. The client talk is unclear about allocating personal and social responsibility: someone needs to act on the chaos, but it is unclear who and by what means.

In sum, the "wish talk" reflects and uses personal responsibility and self-management vocabularies to set recovery aims and visions for the future. The client would want in the future to be self-sufficient and a more active agent, and thus he allies himself with the responsible self at the ideal level. The self-management approach provides a "yardstick" for the client for preferred agency and a vision of a better, more independent future. However, in this example, it does not give means to construct an empowered self who would know how to overcome the barriers in the way of a preferred agency, or who could be helpful in the struggles against dependency. Accordingly, the (mental) chaos is constructed as a force and agent on its own, not managed by the client's endeavours, and it is thus not a question of personal or social responsibility.

Resisting self: accounting for limited responsibility

Limited responsibility due to ...

Next we examine how the clients resist the expectations of personal responsibility and self-management. When the clients formulate resisting accounts, they display their limited abilities and strengths as causes and explanations of why they cannot (try to) live independently without support. The examples illustrate the resistance towards the expectation of personal and social responsibility, the responsible self.

... severe conditions and limited strengths

This example demonstrates a resisting self in a situation where the client's energy and ability to function are limited. The client is from the Finnish floating support service for people with mental health problems. The client is in his twenties. He suffers from severe mental health problems and attention-deficit hyperactivity disorder (ADHD). The interview is conducted in the client's apartment. The extract is from an interview section where client-centredness is discussed.

Extract 3

1   INTERVIEWER: If you think about it, do you have some wishes that you would like to present to the physician, for example, or, what should they take into consideration in your treatment. How should they change their actions?

2   CLIENT: I haven't come up with anything new. Sometimes I feel like there has been too much happening here. I should be doing things all the time, like sorting out and taking care of things and vocational rehabilitation activities and everything. I don't seem to have enough strength for it.

3   INTERVIEWER: What is your role in rehabilitation? What should you do in order to maintain your condition?

4   CLIENT: Well, to live as regularly as possible, regularly, and have a healthy lifestyle. I haven't come up with [anything else]. I'm just trying to make things work in every way I can, to avoid having excessive stress which would make my condition worse.

The extract begins with the interviewer's question concerning the client's wishes for treatment. The question is also formulated to find out the client's view on the welfare workers' roles, possibilities and responsibilities to aid him in managing his condition: is there anything that welfare workers should change in their conduct to be more supportive for the client (turn 1)? The client does not come up with any straightforward requests for the welfare workers, even though the client's response *"sometimes I feel like there has been too much happening here"* can be interpreted to mean that the welfare workers are considered partly responsible for arranging too many things for the client to do. However, the client does not explicitly blame them, but instead blames his limited resources: *"I don't seem to have enough strength for it."* (turn 2). The client interprets his limited strength as a major problem and the one to be blamed. He constructs a cause-and-effect relationship between the feeling of "too much" and a lack of energy. If he had more strength, things would be easier to conduct. Hence, the lack of energy works as an explanation and justification for the client's dif-ficulties in fulfilling the tasks related to a responsible self operating in society and "doing recovery". The client explains that he is struggling to perform the expected tasks at the margins of welfare services, and thus there is the risk that the responsible self is too great a demand in his current situation (turn 2).

The interviewer's second question explicitly addresses personal responsibility and self-management in recovery. It also puts forward a presumption that man-aging mental health requires one to actively do things (turn 3). This may trigger the client to respond by using vocabularies of self-management and by construct-ing recovery as a matter of a particular way of living. He contends that he ought *"to live as regularly as possible, regularly, and have a healthy lifestyle."* In addi-tion, the client explains that he has discovered the importance of avoiding too much stress. In the causal account, the stress is perceived as a cause of the pos-sible worsening of the condition. In other words, sustaining good condition would require circumstances favourable for a life without stress.

In this example, personal responsibility and self-management have been dis-played as demanding activities that would require strong agency and strengths from the client. The client outlines a balance between trying to fulfil the tasks (of the welfare services) and the risk of becoming too stressed. Personal responsib-ility and self-management do not appear as empowering "I talk" or hopeful "wish talk", but as "pressing talk" of things being understood as "too much" and possibly worsening the client's condition. Instead of reaching for more self-management techniques, things to do to manage everyday life, the client tries to avoid increasing activities in life. In this sense, the client talk formulates a crit-ical stance towards the ever-growing demands of personal responsibility and self-management, and it emphasises that they can in some situations work against the liberating aim of becoming an empowered and healthy individual.

... illegitimate/unrealistic expectations

The fourth example is from the supported housing service in England for people with mental health problems. The client is in his thirties and has severe mental health problems. The interview was held in the client's apartment. The data excerpt is from an interview section concerning the client's arrival at the sup-ported housing services.

Extract 4

1 INTERVIEWER: So, if we just talk a bit about your present life here in [supported housing services for people with mental health problems]. So, what do you do with the staff, do you have conversations?

2 CLIENT: Now that I'm moving out, not so much.

3 INTERVIEWER: Oh, that's right.

4 CLIENT: When I first moved in, yeah.

5 INTERVIEWER: You had then.

6 CLIENT: Yeah. When I moved in, yeah, and it's only because I was getting better, better I should say, that it lessened off a little bit, I should say. Check up on me. See if my room was tidy and that. My room's never tidy. My kitchen is. I'll wash the pots, right, and I'll do that, and I actually quite enjoy doing that, right. But my front room is just, it's like a bomb's gone off and I don't know why.

7 INTERVIEWER: So, they come and say to you could you please …

8 CLIENT: Yeah. And I don't do anything. Eventually I'll look at it and think I need to go in the bed now.

9 INTERVIEWER: So, how about discussions, then?

10 CLIENT: Telling a depressed person to do something is really a bad idea.

The extract begins with a question from the interviewer that implies the presumption that using the service comprises encounters and discussions with the workers (turn 1). The client's response constructs the intensity of the client–worker interaction as being bound to the client's well-being and progress in recovery: "*it's only because I was getting better, better I should say, that it lessened off a little bit*" (turn 6). The phrase is a causal account in the sense that "getting better" is seen as a cause for a lessening of the support relationship. It also constructs what the welfare workers do (are responsible for) as part of the support relationship: "*Check up on me. See if my room was tidy*" (turn 6). These activities can be interpreted as worker-led management techniques that have elements of control, ensuring and taking responsibility for the client's coping. The next question-answer sequence (turns 7 and 8) reveals the assumption that the client is directed to eventually internalise the importance of having a tidy room and work for it by himself. The client expresses how he is not acting in accordance with this expectation of a self-managing and personally responsible client: "*My room's never tidy,*" (turn 6), "*I don't do anything. Eventually I'll look at it and think I need to go in the bed now*" (turn 8). The account is a factual statement: it does not indicate that untidiness is a problem for the client or that he would try to change his behaviour in the future. It can be interpreted as resistance towards higher cleanliness standards, more active agency and self-management requirements.

The interviewer goes back to the assumption that a support relationship should include conversations (turn 9). The client responds in an ambiguous way by saying that "*Telling a depressed person to do something is really a bad idea*", which implies that telling someone what to do is not an appropriate technique to approach a person who lacks energy and is depressed (turn 10). The account can thus be read as resistance towards a support relationship that is based on "telling" or advice giving. The turn creates a potential causal account: because the client is "a depressed person", the room is never tidy. Being a depressed person is then put forward as an explanation and justification for the client's passive behaviour. The causal account is constructed in such a way that the situation appears as self-evident, fixed and unchangeable. The account proposes a "fatalistic talk" that there is no means to change a depressed person, and consequently no one is to blame for, or seen as being accountable for, the passive self. It is just a common fact.

... discriminating society

The last example examines social responsibility and society as a context where socially excluded individuals try to manage their lives. The interview interaction does not follow the ordinary pattern of question/answer sequences, as the client both asks the questions and answers them. He uses the question sheet that the interviewer gives to him. In this way, it is easier for the client to stay focused and handle the interview situation. The client was in his thirties and had many special needs related to drug abuse, homelessness, severe mental health conditions and ADHD. The interview was conducted in a Finnish outpatient clinic for people with severe drug abuse problems.

Extract 5

1   CLIENT: Yeah. Yes. Who is responsible for your well-being and recovery? I am, and probably the party treating me. At least on some level. They're responsible for what the treatment is. They're responsible for that at least. I can't really say. How do you see the responsibility or impact of the society regarding your coping or the fact that things haven't always been easy? The society sucks, it tries to put all people into the same category. But when this one person, I'm a Lego piece and I don't belong to that big Lego series. So, I'm flawed and I'm thrown away into the trash can. I'm just a mere nuisance from an elitist point of view.
2   INTERVIEWER: That was a really great analysis. One of the greatest I've ever heard.

The extract begins with the question that the client reads from the question sheet: "*Who is responsible for your well-being and recovery?*" (turn 1), which triggers the client to distribute responsibility between himself and those involved in his care. The client recognises himself as being personally responsible – "*I am*" – and welfare workers as partly responsible for the content of the treatment: "*what the treatment is*" is defined as the scope of the welfare workers' responsibility. The utterance reflects the thought that it is the welfare workers who decide the quantity and quality of treatment services. The client goes on to the next inter-view question, which addresses society's impact on the client's recovery (turn 1). The question gets the client to describe critically how in society there is an attempt to put everyone into the same category and thus not allow for "Lego pieces" that do not belong to the "big Lego series". This metaphor can be under-stood to mean that individuals are grouped into those who are fit for society and those who are not: the outcasts. In addition, it refers to stigmatising, blaming and discriminating societal powers which are beyond the client's control but which do have an influence on his well-being. The client displays how he does not have influence or personal responsibility in society; he is just thrown away by others. The metaphor portrays the client as being "faulty" and "waste" that society does not care for: "*I'm flawed and I'm thrown away into the trash can. I'm just a mere nuisance from an elitist point of view*" (turn 1).

In sum, the data example demonstrates a "drifting talk". It is a description of circumstances that oppress and exploit the self and thus make self-managing dif-ficult. The self is oppressed by powers out of its control and given a degrading position in society. The self is faced with external forces that it is not capable of (or responsible for) taming or turning for the better. The client constructs himself without an entitlement to agency, and thus is at the mercy of others' (discrimi-nating) action. In turn, welfare workers are seen as being only responsible for treatment services. In the example, no one is seen as capable of making a totally inclusive "Lego series" or of taking wider social responsibility: the socially excluded individual's personal responsibility is narrowed to "drifting" and to being an object of the actions of others.

Conclusion and discussions

Much is said about self-responsibility today. Individuals are expected to actively manage their own health and make responsible lifestyle decisions (Roberts 2006; Broom *et al.* 2014). They are supposed to work on themselves and seek expert knowledge in order to learn skills and self-management techniques for better well-being and health (Scott and Wilson 2011; MacGregor and Wathen 2014; Chapter 2 of this volume). In this chapter, we have scrutinised how the clients talk about personal and social responsibility in the process of recovery at the time of rising expectation of self-management and the responsible self (self-responsibilisation). We have illustrated how "theories of causes" are influential and essential in how people construct and distribute responsibility, blame and agency – and thus important matters to examine. Cause construction points to the ones responsible for (exceptional) occasions and life situations (e.g. Pearl and Lebowitz 2014).

We have demonstrated how the clients at the margins of welfare services on the one hand (try to) live up to the ideal of the responsible self, and on the other hand resist this cultural expectation as impossible or unreasonable. They (and interviewers) reflect responsibilities by using client responsibility and the self-management vocabularies. Then they use professional concepts that resonate with the management of health, well-being and life. Self-management vocabularies allow empowering "I talk" and future-oriented, hopeful "wish talk". Clients frequently construct their agency in a way that reflects the ideal individual presented in the era of advanced liberal governance. In other words, they express that they try to be self-sufficient, independent and active in life despite barriers, and it is the "I" that needs to be, and can be, the one that makes the required life changes (see also Chapter 6).

Self-management vocabularies point to individuals' deficiencies that are to be worked on. Thus, it can be interpreted that they trigger "pressing talk" in which recovery activities become constructed as "too much" and a burden according to the client's present strengths and abilities. The self becomes constructed as "insufficient" and "faulty". This way of talking can be seen as the client's linguistic device to resist personal responsibility by stating that limited resources are causing passive agency and a need for support from others. The self-responsibility is an overly demanding expectation in a powerless situation and if *"you're so broken"*.

However, the clients also detach themselves from the self-management approach and personal responsibility by producing resisting "fatalistic talk" that displays their situation as such that there is no means (and no sense) to try to change things for the better or to ease their troubles. Similarly, "drifting talk" positions the client as powerless and oppressed, and thus without the ability to be a personally responsible actor. We conclude that for the clients at the margins of welfare services, managing responsibilities "in action" is a demanding, context-bound and multi-dimensional accomplishment. They are struggling to both be the responsible self with limited resources and detach themselves from this expectation.

Although self-management techniques support clients in managing their everyday lives and offer objectives for more active agency in health and illness, they do not necessarily eliminate the clients' need for support. Personal responsibility is talked into being and reflected in relation to social responsibility. In other words, the clients indicate that in order to take responsibility from themselves, they need to have sufficient resources, and other people such as welfare workers to support and value them. This underscores the relevance of examining further the causal relation constructed between supportive relationships and self-management, as has been already done by previous research (Dashiff 2003; Cramm *et al.* 2015).

Many scholars have claimed that personal and social responsibility are intertwined, related and relational concepts (McNamee and Gergen 1999; Brownell *et al.* 2010; Naumova 2014; Trnka and Trundle 2014). Personal responsibility requires social responsibility: social resources, social support, genuine options in life and reciprocal relations in the community (Brownell *et al.* 2010). Trnka and Trundle (2014: 137) approach the distinction between personal and social responsibility by arguing that responsibilisation contains multiple meanings and needs to be approached not only within an individual neoliberal discourse, but "through the lenses of care relations and social contract ideologies". Similarly, Passini (2011: 284) argues that "the claiming of rights and a sense of duty should always involve the recognition of a responsibility – to oneself as well as to others". Our individual agency is dependent on the actions of others and on our status in the community. There are times when we are able to care for ourselves and others, whilst at other times we might be powerless, helpless and without means to live a meaningful life due to long-term illnesses and adversities.

The clients' talk about recovery and self-responsibility reflects the cultural and moral understanding of what a valued citizen and a valued lifestyle mean (Broom *et al.* 2014; Keddie 2016). We agree with Broom *et al.* (2014: 527) that a cultural norm of duty is to be taken as the core morality implicated in the drive for good health, and that it is also present in advanced liberal governing of the self (see also Brownell *et al.* 2010). Without denying that self-management may promote empowered selves, it can also turn out to be "cruel optimism" for those who do not have the resources or possibilities to achieve positive recovery outcomes by setting them in the position of the ones that fail. MacGregor and Wathen (2014) stress the risk that social determinants are ignored at the political level and "those who cannot manage their own health may fall further behind".

At a time of rising expectations of self-management, clients both try to fulfil the criteria of the responsible self and detach themselves from it. They identify the risk of failures in recovery and the assumed gaps in their life between expectations and actions. Hence, it is critical to work not only on individual conduct but also on the cause-and-effect relation in play and "relational re-responsibilisation". The relevant questions are: how is valued and "sufficiently" responsible agency culturally constructed? Whose responsibility is it to promote and support this agency? The responsible self is a reciprocal, social, relational and negotiable construction, and is thus a collective accomplishment.

References

Antaki, C. (1994) *Explaining and Arguing: The social organization of accounts*, London: Sage.
Ballet, J., Dubois, J.-L. and Mahieu, F.-R. (2007) "Responsibility for each other's freedom: agency as the source of collective capability", *Journal of Human Development*, 8(2): 185–201.
Beckmann, N. (2013) "Responding to medical crises: AIDS treatment, responsibilisation and the logic of choice", *Anthropology & Medicine*, 20(2): 160–174.
Broom, A., Meurk, C., Adams, J. and Sibbritt, D. (2014) "My health, my responsibility? Complementary medicine and self (health) care", *Journal of Sociology*, 50(4): 515–530.
Brownell, K.D., Kersh, R., Ludwig, D.S., Post, R.C., Puhl, R.M., Schwartz, M.B. and Willett, W.C. (2010) "Personal responsibility and obesity: a constructive approach to a controversial issue", *Health Affairs*, 29(3): 379–87.
Bull, R. and Shaw, I. (1992) "Constructing causal accounts in social work", *Sociology*, 26(4): 635–649.
Buttny, R. (1993) *Social Accountability in Communication*, London: Sage.
Cappelen, A.W. and Norheim, O.F. (2005) "Responsibility in health care: a liberal egalitarian approach", *Journal of Medical Ethics*, 31(8): 476–480.

Cayton, H. (2006) "The flat-pack patient? Creating health together", *Patient Education and Counseling*, 62(3): 288–290.

Civaner, M. and Arda, B. (2008) "Do patients have responsibilities in a free market system? A personal perspective", *Nursing Ethics*, 15(2): 263–273.

Clarke, J. (2005) "New Labour's citizens: activated, empowered, responsibilized, abandoned?", *Critical Social Policy*, 25(4): 447–463.

Cole, J., Logan, T.K. and Walker, R. (2011) "Social exclusion, personal control, self-regulation, and stress among substance abuse treatment clients", *Drug & Alcohol Dependence*, 113(1): 13–20.

Cramm, J., Murray, N. and Anna, P. (2015) "Chronically ill patients' self-management abilities to maintain overall well-being: what is needed to take the next step in the primary care setting?", *BMC Family Practice*, 16(1): 1–8.

Cruikshank, B. (1996) "Revolutions within: self-government and self-esteem", in A. Barry, T. Osborne and N. Rose (eds) *Foucault and Political Reason: Liberalism, neo-liberalism and rationalities of government* (pp. 231–252), Chicago: University of Chicago Press.

Dashiff, C.J. (2003) "Self- and dependent-care responsibility of adolescents with IDDM and their parents", *Journal of Family Nursing*, 9(2): 166–183.

Davidson, L. (2005) "Recovery, self management and the expert patient: changing the culture of mental health from a UK perspective", *Journal of Mental Health*, 14(1): 25–35.

Dean, M. (2002) "Liberal government and authoritarianism", *Economy and Society*, 31(1): 37–61.

Dickens, G., Weleminsky, J., Onifade, Y. and Sugarman, P. (2012) "Recovery Star: validating user recovery", *The Psychiatrist*, 36: 45–50, DOI: 10.1192/pb.bp. 111.034264.

Doheny, S. (2007) "Responsibility and the deliberative citizen: theorizing the acceptance of individual and citizenship responsibilities", *Citizenship Studies*, 11(4): 405–420.

Doughty, C., Tse, S., Duncan, N. and McIntyre, L. (2008) "The Wellness Recovery Action Plan (WRAP): workshop evaluation", *Australasian Psychiatry*, 16(6): 450–456.

Edwards, D. and Potter, J. (1993) "Language and causation: a discursive action model of description and attribution", *Psychological Review*, 100(1): 23–41.

Flynn, D. (2005) "What's wrong with rights? Rethinking human rights and responsibilities", *Australian Social Work*, 58(3): 244–256.

Garfinkel, H. (1967) *Studies in Ethnomethodology*, Cambridge: Polity Press.

Giddens, A. (1999) "Risk and responsibility", *The Modern Law Review*, 62(1): 1–10.

Hazleden, B. (2014) "Whose fault is it? Exoneration and allocation of personal responsibility in relationship manual", *Journal of Sociology*, 50(4): 422–436.

Holen, M. and Ahrenkiel, A. (2011) " 'After all, you should rather want to be at home': responsibility as a means to patient involvement in the Danish health system", *Journal of Social Work Practice: Psychotherapeutic approaches in health, welfare and the community*, 25(3): 297–310.

Ilcan, S. (2009) "Privatizing responsibility: public sector reform under neoliberal government", *Canadian Review of Sociology*, 46(3): 207–234.

Jallinoja, P., Absetz, P., Kuronen, R., Nissinen, A., Talja, M., Uutela, A. and Patja, K. (2007) "The dilemma of patient responsibility for lifestyle change: perceptions among primary care physicians and nurses", *Scandinavian Journal of Primary Health Care*, 25(4): 244–249.

Johnston, S., Liddy, C., Ives, S.M. and Soto, E. (2008) *Literature Review on Chronic Disease Self-Management*, retrieved 10 December 2015 from www.livinghealthy champlain.ca/documents/pages/ReviewChronicDisease.pdf.

Juhila, K., Hall, C. and Raitakari, S. (2010) "Accounting for the clients' troublesome behaviour in a supported housing unit: blames, excuses and responsibility in professionals' talk", *Journal of Social Work*, 10(1): 59–79.

Keddie, A. (2015) "New modalities of state power: neoliberal responsibilisation and the work of academy chains", *International Journal of Inclusive Education*, 19(11): 1190–1205.

Kelty, C.M. (2008) "Responsibility: McKeon and Ricoeur", *Anthropology of the Contemporary Research Collaboratory*, Working Paper #12, retrieved 10 December 2015 from http://kelty.org/or/papers/Kelty-Mckeon-Ricoeur-WP12.pdf.

Lister, M. (2015) "Citizens, doing it for themselves? The Big Society and government through community", *Parliamentary Affairs*, 68(2): 352–370.

Lorig, K. and Holman, H.R. (2003) "Self management education: history, definition, outcomes, and mechanisms", *Annals of Behavioral Medicine*, 26(1): 1–7.

Lorig, K., Holman, H., Sobel, D., Laurent, D., González, V. and Minor, M. (1994) *Living a Healthy Life with Chronic Conditions*, Palo Alto, CA: Bull Publishing Company.

Lundell, H., Niederdeppe, J. and Clarke, C. (2013) "Public views about health causation, attributions of responsibility, and inequality", *Journal of Health Communication*, 18(9): 1116–1130.

Lyon-Callo, V. (2000) "Medicalizing homelessness: the production of self-blame and self-governing within homeless shelters", *Medical Anthropology Quarterly*, 14(3): 328–345.

MacGregor, J.C.D. and Wathen, C.N. (2014) " 'My health is not a job': a qualitative exploration of personal health management and imperatives of the 'new public health' ", *BMC Public Health*, 14(1): 726–735.

Matarese, M. and Caswell, D. (2014) "Accountability", in C. Hall, K. Juhila, M. Matarese and C. Van Nijnatten (eds) *Analysing Social Work Communication: Discourse in practice* (pp. 44–60), London: Routledge.

May, J., Carey, T.A. and Curry, R. (2013) "Social determinants of health: whose responsibility?", *Australian Journal of Rural Health*, 21(3): 139–140.

McNamee, S. and Gergen, K.J. (1999) *Relational Responsibility: Resources for sustainable dialogue*, London: Sage.

Michailakis, D. and Schirmer, W. (2010) "Agents of their health? How the Swedish welfare state introduces expectations of individual responsibility", *Sociology of Health and Illness*, 32(6): 930–947.

Miller, P. and Rose, N. (2008) *Governing the Present: Administering economic, social and personal life*, Cambridge: Polity Press.

Naumova, E.N. (2014) "A cautionary note for population health: disproportionate emphasis on personal responsibility for health and wellbeing", *Journal of Public Health Policy*, 35(3): 397–400.

Onifade, Y. (2011) "The mental health recovery star", *Mental Health and Social Inclusion*, 15(2): 78–87.

Passini, S. (2011) "Individual responsibilities and moral inclusion in an age of rights", *Culture & Psychology*, 17(3): 281–296.

Pearl, R.L. and Lebowitz, M.S. (2014) "Beyond personal responsibility: effects of causal attributions for overweight and obesity on weight-related beliefs, stigma, and policy support", *Psychology & Health*, 29(10): 1176–1191.

Pulvirenti, M., McMillan, J. and Lawn, S. (2014) "Empowerment, patient centered care and self-management", *Health Expectations*, 17(3): 303–310.

Raitakari, S., Günther, K., Juhila, K. and Saario, S. (2013) "Causal accounts as a consequential device in categorizing mental health and substance abuse problems", *Communication & Medicine*, 10(3): 237–248.

Robert, S.A., Booske, B.C., Rigby, E. and Rohan, A.M. (2008) "Public views on determinants of health, interventions to improve health, and priorities for government", *Wisconsin Medical Journal*, 107(3): 124–130.

Roberts, C. (2006) "'What can I do to help myself?' Somatic individuality and contemporary hormonal bodies", *Science Studies*, 19(2): 54–76.

Rose, N. (1990) *Governing the Soul: The shaping of the private self*, London: Routledge.

Rose, N. (1996) "The death of the social? Re-figuring the territory of government", *Economy and Society*, 25(3): 327–356.

Scott, M. and Lyman, S. (1968) "Accounts", *American Sociological Review*, 33(1): 46–62.

Scott, A. and Wilson, L. (2011) "Valued identities and deficit identities: Wellness Recovery Action Planning and self-management in mental health", *Nursing Inquiry*, 18(1): 40–49.

Share, M. and Strain, M. (2008) "Making schools and young people responsible: a critical analysis of Ireland's obesity strategy", *Health & Social Care in the Community*, 16(3): 234–243.

Snelling, P.C. (2012) "Saying something interesting about responsibility for health", *Nursing Philosophy*, 13(3): 161–178.

Social Exclusion Unit (2004) *Tackling Social Exclusion: Taking stock and looking to the future, emerging findings*, London: Office of the Deputy Prime Minister.

Solberg, J. (2011) "Accepted and resisted: the client's responsibility for making proposals in activation encounters", *Text & Talk*, 31(6): 733–752.

Stasiulis, D. and Bakan, A. (2003) *Negotiating Citizenship: Migrant women in Canada and the global system*, New York: Palgrave Macmillan.

Sterling, E.W., von Esenwein, S.A., Tucker, S., Fricks, L. and Druss, B.G. (2010) "Integrating wellness, recovery, and self-management for mental health consumers", *Community Mental Health Journal*, 46(2): 130–138.

Tickle, A., Cheung, N. and Walker, C. (2013) "Professionals' perceptions of the Mental Health Recovery Star", *Mental Health Review Journal*, 18(4): 194–203.

Trnka, S. and Trundle, C. (2014) "Competing responsibilities: moving beyond neoliberal responsibilisation", *Anthropological Forum: A Journal of Social Anthropology and Comparative Sociology*, 24(2): 136–153.

van Houtum, L., Rijken, M. and Groenewegen, P. (2015) "Do everyday problems of people with chronic illness interfere with their disease management?", *BMC Public Health*, 15(1): 1–9.

Wikler, D. (2002) "Personal and social responsibility for health", *Ethics & International Affairs*, 16(2): 47–56.

Wiley, L.F., Berman, M.L. and Blanke, D. (2013) "Who's your nanny?: Choice, paternalism and public health in the age of personal responsibility", *Journal of Law, Medicine & Ethics*, Supplement 41: 88–91.

6 Making active citizens in the community in client–worker interaction

Suvi Raitakari and Nichlas Permin Berger

Introduction

Vulnerable citizens are increasingly supported, treated and regulated in the community, in normal housing and in neighbourhoods. Inclusion and normal life in the community are also often an individual's first priority and wish (Sayce 2000; Davidson *et al.* 2001; Padfield and Maruna 2006). This "return to the community" has been due to the major deinstitutionalisation process launched in the Western world during recent decades, which has resulted in a reduction in institutional services and an increase in home- and community-based services: a shift of professional support and control from institutions to the community. The transformation process is supported by human rights (a move from institutional-professional control to increasing self-determination and self-management), cost saving and recovery arguments (Fakhoury and Priebe 2002; Priebe *et al.* 2005; Ramon 2008; Davidson *et al.* 2010).

Those citizens who experience severe mental difficulties and those who have to deal with the criminal justice system are among the most vulnerable and stigmatised people in our society (Hartwell 2004). They commonly face great challenges in the re-entry process from institutional care or prison to the community due to the common and complex concurrence of substance abuse, mental difficulties, unemployment, homelessness and discrimination (Sayce 2000, 2003; Hartwell 2004; Serin *et al.* 2010: 62; Rowe and Baranoski 2011). As Turner (2012: 322) states, "the prisoner is often determined as the 'other' and at a distance, metaphorical as well as physical, from the citizen majority". Isolation, (self-)stigmatisation, poverty, loneliness and a lack of fitting education and work are common experiences among vulnerable citizens. They do not easily experience belonging and membership in the community (Amado *et al.* 2013: 360; Turner 2012). Full citizenship and life in the community is thus a struggle for vulnerable citizens, and requires resilience and resistance against discrimination and social exclusion (Sayce 2000; Mezzina *et al.* 2006a; Rowe and Baranoski 2011; Ponce *et al.* 2012; Hamer *et al.* 2014).

This hardship of living in the community highlights the need for adequate community-based support and treatment services (Davidson *et al.* 2001; Serin *et al.* 2010: 62). For example, a home visit is often a preferred community-based working technique to enhance vulnerable citizens' everyday life in "normal" settings such as homes, public venues and social events. Also, different representatives from prison, probation, police, (mental) health and social services, together with the client, are expected to plan, coordinate and implement the provision and delivery of a range of services and programmes to support citizens' successful return from the institutional setting to the communal one (Frazier *et al.* 2015).

Successful return to the community is linked in political, academic and professional discussions to active citizenship and participation (e.g. Turner 2012). Living in the community is seen to require active membership in local networks in work, study and leisure (Rose 1996). Active citizenship and participation thus implies an ideal and recovered individual. In this chapter, we scrutinise how the discourse of active citizenship is reflected and resisted in client–worker interaction in mental health home visits and in prison pre-release conferences. By a close analysis of the data, we demonstrate how workers construct clients as active and responsible members of the community and how clients contribute to or resist this making of an active citizen. Making active citizens is shown to be based on the specific working techniques: (1) planning, (2) questioning, (3) going along, (4) coaching and (5) networking. Before the data examples, we introduce active citizenship discourse and how it interprets participation, recovery and risk related to the idea of the "return to the community". Both enabling and coercive meanings embedded in the discourse are described. It is discussed especially how the discourse constructs division between an "active citizen" and a "non-active citizen" and thus justifies the workers' efforts to strengthen and govern clients' abilities to be active members of the community. We argue that citizens – especially those who confront the task of re-entering the community from institutional care and control settings – are governed by the requirement to become active and responsible members of the community.

Active citizenship as enabling and coercive discourse

Government through community

"Government through community" and the active citizenship discourse are at the centre of political and academic attention in the Western world (Rose 1996; Ilcan and Basok 2004; Schinkel and van Houdt 2010; Staeheli 2013: 522). Within the active citizenship discourse, community is constructed as a pivotal locality to govern and perform citizenship. As Pathak (2013: 62) states, "[in Britain] attempts to responsibilise citizens are reciprocal and concurrent with the promotion, production and reformation of communities as relational spaces for the performance of active citizenship". The community is constructed as an arena for promoting and regulating political, civic and consumer participation (Eriksson 2012; Pathak 2013: 70). In other words, the discourse comprises two meanings: personal participation and responsibility in the community; and the community as the locality in which to perform, carry out and govern citizenship

(Rose 1996; Schinkel and van Houdt 2010: 697; Turner 2012: 322). In addition, the active citizenship discourse comprises debates on "whether citizenship is about the rights which flow to citizens or on the obligations which citizens have to their society" (Bolzan and Gale 2002: 365). In this chapter, active citizenship is approached as the culturally expected end result of vulnerable citizens' personal participation, recovery and responsibility in the community.

The active citizenship discourse can be approached as an enabling discourse that indicates various empowering pre-assumptions such as freedom, independence and choice-making; along with participation, integration, inclusion and involvement in services, the community and one's life (Bolzan and Gale 2002). Ilcan and Basok (2004: 132) formulate this enabling side of governmentality through active citizenship discourse in the following way (see also Rose 1996):

> In fact, it can be said that the task of government today is no longer engaged in traditional planning but is more involved in enabling, inspiring, and assisting citizens to take responsibility for social problems in their community, and formulating appropriate orientations and rationalities for their actions.

However, the discourse is simultaneously coercive by defining those who are seen as not fulfilling the obligations of being active citizens for subjects of re-responsibilisation and re-integration (see Chapter 2). Jauffret-Roustide (2009: 169), who studied drug users' social movements and struggles to regain citizenship in France, states: "The meaning of self-reliance, responsibility, citizenship and patients' expertise can also be the product of professional and militant constructions". In other words, the active citizenship discourse embeds a coercive-moralising dimension, and thus it enables making the divisions between "good" and "competent" citizens and those who are not.

Participation, recovery and risk

The intent of the active citizenship discourse is to govern citizens by setting the norm of what it means to be an acceptable individual. It puts forwards normative views on responsible citizens and how they should relate to each other (Schinkel and van Houdt 2010; Staeheli 2013: 524). Citizens ought to be independent, self-controlled and able to participate in activities in their neighbourhoods, self-care groups, voluntary work, studying and working (Pols 2006: 98; Chapter 2 of this volume). Citizens are expected to be self-reliant and morally responsible, i.e. to take care of themselves and others (Ramon 2008). Active citizenship is about supporting, integrating and looking after oneself and others. The discourse implies, therefore, obligations and respected social roles in a community setting (Staeheli 2013; Bee and Pachi 2014). Accordingly, one consequence of the active citizenship discourse is that it creates demarcation of those who are able to take full responsibility in the community from those who cannot. "Non-active" citizens are politically and morally undervalued as being the opposite of active citizens (Rose 1996; Kemshall 2002).

The discourse reconstructs relations between citizens, the third sector, the (welfare) state and the market in a way that justifies the decreasing of public welfare and the increasing of citizens' responsibility for taking care of themselves and others (Ilcan and Basok 2004; Ilcan 2009; Schinkel and van Houdt 2010: 669–670; Staeheli 2013: 522). The active citizenship discourse turns the gaze to individual citizens as the source of welfare. It "implies freedom, but it is a freedom through which the government of individuals and populations is made possible" (Perron *et al.* 2010: 106).

When the discourse is translated and adopted by specific fields such as mental health, substance abuse, homelessness, probation and youth work (e.g. Rowe *et al.* 2001; Milbourne 2009; Perron *et al.* 2010), it is understood positively in relation to recovery and the importance of being a member of a local community such as in family relationships, self-help groups and educational and leisure activity groups (e.g. Mezzina *et al.* 2006a, 40; Sells *et al.* 2006; Rose and Baranowski 2011). For instance, Rowe *et al.* (2001: 15) argue that "the concept of 'citizenship' provides a useful framework for addressing the challenge of linking mentally ill homeless persons to their communities". They define citizenship as a "measure of the strength of people's connection to the rights, responsibilities, roles, and resources that society offers to people through public and social institutions and to relationships involving close ties, supportive social networks, and associational life in one's community" (see also Rowe and Baranoski 2011: 304; Rowe and Pelletier 2012: 368).

In mental health work, citizenship is especially approached as a precondition and consequence of recovery (e.g. Mezzina *et al.* 2006b: 80; Davidson *et al.* 2010*)*. It is emphasised that the community can both promote yet also disallow the process of becoming an active citizen in the community. Unsupportive, stigmatising and disrespectful relations and a lack of resources may hinder recovery and increase mental health difficulties. A person becomes a citizen through interaction in the community. Recovery is then defined as a process during which dependence on others decreases and capacity to contribute to the well-being of others increases (Topor *et al.* 2006; Mezzina *et al.* 2006b). As Rowe and Pelletier (2012: 379) put it: "A large part of what is to be 'recovered' or achieved, we argue, is one's citizenship".

When the active citizenship discourse is adopted into the field of criminal justice, it is translated more as a restoration of the moral duties and rights of criminals through re-integrative practices that strengthen democracy (Uggen *et al.* 2006). In addition, active citizenship is understood as a precondition and a consequence of self-responsibilisation (Kemshall 2002; Aharonson and Ramsay 2010; Turner 2012). Researchers (e.g. Garland 2001; Rose 2002; O'Malley 2010; Goddard 2012) in the field of criminal justice have applied and developed the ideas of responsibilisation techniques and practices of the neoliberal states. Prison and probation officers' punitive and risk (assessment) based working practices may increasingly be seen to strive to make active citizens who are able to re-enter the community. This is often attempted through increasing the inmates' awareness of the risk thinking and their own risk/need factors (e.g.

Turnbull and Hannah-Moffat 2009). It is argued that in the field of criminal justice, notions of risk permeate institutional practices and constitute subjectivities that possess risk thinking.

Generally, risk is connected with neoliberal regulatory strategies that emphasise self-sufficiency, responsibility and empowerment as essential characteristics of preferred citizenship (Rose 2000; Bosworth 2007; Turnbull and Hannah-Moffat 2009). Conceiving crime as an individual choice means that prosocial choices are seen as a necessary means of exercising one's freedom. As put by Hardy (2014: 307), "Under 'risk', the aim is to produce reasonable, autonomous and 'risk-free' individuals". Risk thinking and the aim to constitute self-governing subjects are embedded in the active citizenship discourse, although it also comprises more empowering and liberating meanings of participation and recovery in the community.

The active citizenship discourse has been criticised for being exclusionary: constructing divisions between "productive" and "non-productive" citizens. Critics argue that the active citizen discourse blames the victims and individualises social risks and inequalities (Eriksson 2012; Chapter 2 of this volume). It also endorses coercive governing practices that are justified by the pursuit of transforming "risky" persons into "non-risky" ones. Next, we will illustrate how workers in their everyday practices construct clients as active citizens and how clients respond to these constructions. In the analysis we utilise both an enabling and a critical reading of the active citizenship discourse.

Making active members in the community

The starting point for the analysis is that the active citizenship discourse as a manifestation of governmentality is present in the grass-roots level practices, and in particular working techniques (e.g. planning) and client categorisations (e.g. portraying the client as one who ought to overcome the barriers to enter public venues and events). Within the discourse, it is believed that passive citizens are in need of special support, education, disciplining and training to become active citizens in the community. Mental health research introduces practical techniques by which clients and workers accomplish active citizenship (see Mezzina *et al.* 2006b; Pols 2006; Davidson *et al.* 2010). This line of research borrows from Rose's (1996: 328) definition of governmentality: "the deliberations, strategies, tactics and devices employed by authorities for making up and acting upon a population and its constituents to ensure good and avert ill" (see also Dean 2002; Pathak 2013: 63; Hazleden 2014; see Chapter 1 of this volume). Rose (1990) uses the term "technology of citizenship" to denote a strategy or technique that aims at the transformation of subjectivity from powerlessness to active citizenship (see also Hazleden 2014: 423; Chapter 5 of this volume). This chapter relates to this research branch.

In the next section, common working techniques are described and analysed that aim to enhance clients' integration into the community. The sub-sections are titled according to these working techniques. The chosen data examples illustrate how the worker and the client construct, negotiate, resist and struggle with the client categories and responsibilities of an active citizen. By close reading, we show how subtle client categorisation is done to enable the shift from "non-active" to "active" citizen. The related question of who is responsible for a successful integration is also focused on. Clients and workers in mental health and prisons often approach active citizenship as a conditional category. It is thought to be achieved by self-management and adopting personal and social responsibilities in the community (e.g. Pols 2006; Hamer *et al.* 2014; Chapter 5 of this volume).

Planning: aiming at active citizenship

The first example[1] is from a Finnish supported housing and floating support service for people with mental health and substance abuse problems. Worker–client interaction takes place in a case-planning meeting involving a worker from the service and the client. The following excerpts are from various parts of such a meeting, which lasted 40 minutes. They illustrate the tone of the whole conversation.

The worker opens the meeting by reading out the recovery aims documented in the client's care plan. The plan contains such aims as adapting to a substance-free way of life, accepting his mental illness, participating in recovery activities organised by the service and attending Alcoholics Anonymous (AA) group gatherings. The worker does not openly blame the client, but the client immediately responds to the opening by saying that he wants to comment on the realisation of these aims. He reflects that the realisation has been unsuccessful. He confesses that he has not been able to increase his participation in the proposed activities. The data example demonstrates how planning and checking on the realisation of recovery aims is one way to govern the transformation from "non-active" to "active" citizen.

Extract 1

1 CLIENT: I'm the kind that gets going pretty slowly.
2 WORKER: Yes. You need some time.
3 CLIENT: I do need a bit of time and ...
4 WORKER: To internalise things.
5 CLIENT: I've had this wish for myself that I've set for myself that I could attend the AA groups even in the evening. I mean weekdays, because I haven't managed to go. The Sunday group has been the one that I've managed to attend.
    [The discussion continues by stating that it is easier for the client to attend a self-help group if it is in the daytime and it is not dark outside. Also, alcohol use and how the client needs to put up with bad feelings and mental health symptoms in his everyday life are addressed, along with the importance of being among other people.]

6   CLIENT: But I can't set a definite day for it. See, my own state of mind is such that I can't set a permanent, like I can't set myself a definite day except Sunday. It just depends so much on what my state of mind is. How I feel, as to whether I can attend a group or not.

7   WORKER: It just crossed my mind. I can't remember who it was that said this, that you are able to go no matter what your feelings are, whatever it is, you could attend a group.

8   CLIENT: So you mean you could go.

   [The worker confirms that the client should try to attend a group although he has difficult feelings. The client describes how anxiety and stress are new experiences for him and how they restrict his activity. He explains how he has heard voices for seven years and has got used to them.]

9   CLIENT: I can cope with everyday things all right. But if it's decisions to do with the future …

10   WORKER: You mean it's somehow difficult for you to think about that, to get a grip?

11   CLIENT: It is, to get a grip on things. I do have this difficulty with thinking. In fact, what I can manage is to wake up in the morning and plan my day, the programme, and then try to get through it. So that's what it's like for me now, just a day at a time.

12   WORKER: You mean it needs to be very concrete and a day at a time.

13   CLIENT: That I can manage.

14   WORKER: So if it is too abstract you can't do it.

15   CLIENT: Making a weekly programme, like, I just couldn't do it. I mean thinking ahead a whole week.

   [The client explains how he has no strength to overcome bad feelings and to attend groups. The client and the worker also discuss how the forthcoming intoxicant treatment will probably also include groups and require active work on oneself.]

16   WORKER: So it's good that you have these regular things in your week that you always do and decide to participate in, no matter how you feel. It's, that's precisely the rehearsing and learning.

At the beginning of the extract the client and the worker jointly categorise the client as not that active (turns 1–4). This "slow person" client categorisation is shared and accepted by both participants, and it is depicted as an explanation for why the client does not attend activities he wishes to (evening AA groups). The objective of being the expected active citizen can be read from the client's fifth turn and its conditional format, "wish talk". The client longs to be more active and to attend the self-help group more often, but (for now) it is impossible for him. The active citizenship is subordinated by an unpredictable and changeable state of mind, "*how I feel*" (turn 6). The client explains and justifies his "passivity" by his unreliable state of mind, which causes uncertainty and difficulties in planning and knowing beforehand what can be accomplished the following day.

The client portrays himself as being controlled by his changing state of mind and feelings (turn 6).

The worker resists this "drifting", not self-governing client categorisation in a subtle manner by using the voice of an expert: *"you are able to go no matter what your feelings are, whatever it is, you could attend a group"* (turn 7). This indirect and not very confrontational account can be interpreted in many ways. It can be seen as advice that attempts to direct the client's conduct towards active citizenship and empowerment as well as to give encouragement for recovery, i.e. that it is possible for the client to improve his level of functioning despite his difficulties.

The client continues depicting himself as a person who lives one day at a time, and in this way he sees himself as managing with *"everyday things all right"* (turn 9). Yet he recognises that he has difficulties in meeting the expectations of an active citizen who is a future-oriented, life-planning decision-maker: *"But if it's decisions to do with the future or ..."* (turn 9); *"I do have this difficulty with thinking"* (turn 11); *"Making a weekly programme, like, I just couldn't do it. I mean thinking ahead a whole week"* (turn 15).

Interestingly, the worker and the client jointly construct and accept the categorisation of the "stagnant" client. Yet, the worker simultaneously also resists this portrayal of a "non-active" client. At the end of the extract, the worker prompts and advocates participation and self-determined behaviour. Active citizenship becomes interpreted as something that can be achieved by *"rehearsing and learning"* (turn 15) through the client's individual endeavours. Responsibility for achieving the desired behaviour is therefore handed over to the client himself. By defining regularity, determination and participation as preferred features, the worker also implies active citizenship as a morally desirable client category.

In summary, the worker recognises his responsibility for building up recovery-friendly, supportive and encouraging interaction. He also carries out the duty to empower the client by assuring the client that he can live out his wishes despite the difficulties. Yet, by simultaneously "forcing" the client to reflect on his failures, the worker is setting the norms and expectations of an active citizenship. The client's current "stagnant" life situation becomes defined in the interaction as problematic (although also understandable in the current situation). The worker is using planning, assessment, advice-giving and supervising techniques to direct the client towards desirable active citizenship, which requires self-government and involvement in the community.

For his part, the client displays responsible citizenship by confessing that his current conduct is not meeting the recovery expectations. Nevertheless, the client also resists the citizenship discourse by describing how he cannot govern the unpredictable mind. Thus, in the interaction there is a pull between an "active" and a "non-active" citizen. A critical question is: when is it justifiable to be passive and to live in the moment, and when should welfare workers be responsible for directing clients to become more active citizens in the community?

Questioning: prompting for social citizenship

The second example[2] is from a Finnish floating support service for people with mental health problems. The interaction takes place on a regular home visit.

Extract 2

1 WORKER: How about going to the grocery store or things like that? Have you visited any store with [boyfriend's name] or a flea market, to be around other people?

2 CLIENT: Last weekend we did go somewhere. [Boyfriend's name] has been working quite a lot, or he has been repairing cars, so he has dropped by somewhere on the way home.

3 WORKER: Have you had any energy to keep in contact with friends?

4 CLIENT: Through the internet. Because it's easy.

5 WORKER: Yes, but you haven't visited anyone or invited anyone to your place?

6 CLIENT: No. You can't really invite anyone here.

7 WORKER: So did you consider that if you could change the room and the arrangements, you could then do that?

[The discussion continues by the client explaining how her boyfriend is planning to invite his friends over, but it is uncertain if the plan will come to fruition.]

Noteworthy in this extract is the way the worker's questioning prompts for the shift from "non-active" to "active" citizen. What kind of activities and behaviour are associated with being an active citizen can be seen from the questions concerning the client's everyday activities and pursuits. The worker's first turn, a three-question series, displays the expectations and requirements of an active citizen: you are supported to be able to get out of the apartment and enter into public places, to take care of your everyday matters and to socialise. The worker's questions indicate that the client has (had) difficulties in accomplishing this "basic level" citizenship, and the client becomes categorised in the interaction as potentially withdrawing and reclusive.

The client responds by first denying the depiction of a recluse: "*Last weekend we did go somewhere*". And second by giving an excuse: "*[Boyfriend's name] has been working quite a lot, or he has been repairing cars, so he has dropped by somewhere on the way home*" (turn 2). For the client, there has not been the need or the possibility to get out of the apartment. In this way the client resists the worker's assumption that there is a problem of her not being sufficiently active.

The worker turns to another aspect of active citizenship, i.e. being social (turn 3). Again the intervention is done through asking a question that comprises an implication of a potential problem (the client being "antisocial"). The client partly accepts this negative categorisation as she responds: "*Through the internet. Because it's easy*" (turn 4). From the worker's response (turn 5), another candidate accusation can be read, namely that being in contact with people via the internet is not sufficient sociality and does not solely meet the criteria of an active citizen. The client admits that she has not been social in this expected way. She defends her "failure" by indicating that the home is not in a suitable condition for having guests (turn 6). The worker replies with a question that comprises a suggestion and advice (turn 7). It also formulates a message that such barriers concerning the home space are removable.

As a whole, the example shows how the worker is taking the responsibility for directing the interaction, as well as for setting the (moral) criteria for proper sociality via asking questions. The client's justifications and excuses can be interpreted as a subtle way to resist the suspicion of her being "non-active" and "antisocial". The questioning implies what kind of social activities the client ought to reach for in her recovery process, i.e. becoming a full citizen. But the questions are not just questions: they set forth moral expectations and preferred client categorisations. Thus, questioning is an important technique in supporting and directing clients' actions. Questioning has empowering potential, because it gives the client a possibility to voice and explain his/her conduct and reality. It is also a way for the worker to show interest in the client's functioning and well-being. Questioning often includes indirect advice that is a delicate way to make an intervention and point to deficiencies in the client's life. However, it can be critically asked how helpful (moral) questioning is for vulnerable citizens with scarce resources and strengths.

Going along: strengthening mobile citizenship

The third example is a discussion between a worker and a client in an English supported housing and floating support service for people with mental health problems. At first, the discussion takes place in the client's home, and later on a walk in the neighbourhood. The main purpose for the home visits is to enable the client to overcome his fear of walking to the town and in the neighbourhood. He has difficulties in getting out of the apartment, and when he does he only walks in a very limited area. There are particular streets and landmarks that he is not able to pass.

Extract 3

1 WORKER: Would you find it personally easier if you progressed with staff rather than being asked to do it on your own?
2 CLIENT: I like the idea of being, I think I need the staff as well. I still need that because you need to get me into the town and I won't be able to do that. But all I can do is me ... gradually, like, do, where we've been on my own to see if I can use my techniques as well. But I need you first of all to get me into there. There's no way I could do that on my own.

3   WORKER: Well that's…. As an end result it's not saying you've got a week to do it.

4   CLIENT: Yeah. I know, yeah.

5   WORKER: As far as we're concerned, if it takes six months it takes six months. We're not going to pressure you.

6   CLIENT: Yeah. That's right.

7   WORKER: It's whatever you feel comfortable with.

8   CLIENT: Oh, right. That's fine, yeah.

9   WORKER: The main thing is getting there in the end.

10   CLIENT: Definitely, yeah. Oh, definitely. That's the main goal.

11   WORKER: So don't ever feel under pressure from us. You just go.

12   CLIENT: Right, yes. That's fine, yeah.

   [The discussion continues with the worker asking for the client's contact information and service contacts. Then the client and the worker get ready to go for a walk and talk about sports. In the section below, the client and worker are walking outside.]

13   WORKER: Well, that's it. Yeah. So, as far as our visits are concerned. Once we start to get further and further, hopefully, is there anything in particular you would like to do?

14   CLIENT: I see what you mean. Yeah.

15   WORKER: Could be something simple as just going for a coffee or …

16   CLIENT: I was going to say.

17   WORKER: Get a bun or whatever.

18   CLIENT: Yeah. You mean once we've hit the town?

19   WORKER: Yeah.

20   CLIENT: Yeah. I think my goal after that is then is for me [unclear] I have to be in and out. I don't like to. I can't do. I don't like to just look around. I have to be bang, in, out, get my stuff, get back into my own place.

The worker asks the client to consider if the workers' plan is relevant for him in order to reach the aim of walking to the town (turn 1). The client constructs himself as dependent on the workers' support and gives them the mandate "*to get me into the town*" (turn 2). Yet, he also emphasises that finally he has to manage to do it "*on my own*" (turn 2). He depicts himself as active and "trying" yet needing the support of the workers. The workers are given a task to take the client out and "push" him into being a mobile citizen in the neighbourhood.

   The worker approaches the recovery task as demanding and time consuming (turns 3 and 5), thereby lessening the pressure on the client to accomplish quick recovery results, i.e. to be in the near future a mobile, self-reliant citizen. The workers have time and understanding for slow progress, and the client is given the right to take gradual steps: "*As far as we're concerned, if it takes six months it takes six months*" (turn 5). The time taken is not that important as long as the client is able to go to the town by himself; "*the main thing is getting there in the end*" (turn 9).

The worker continues by giving the client an opportunity to make choices and express preferences and wishes. He also depicts a positive image of recovery: "*Once we start to get further and further, hopefully, is there anything in particular you would like to do?*" (turn 13). The worker's responses can be interpreted as attempts to strengthen the category of a choice-maker and a competent citizen. The client grasps the idea of himself spending time at public venues in the future (turn 14), but does not expect a total transformation in his conduct: "*I have to be bang, in, out, get my stuff, get back into my own place*" (turn 20). Although he would "*hit the town*" (turn 18*)* and thus meet the recovery aim, there would still potentially be deficiencies and difficulties for him to be mobile and a public citizen (turn 20). However, the client depicts his activity also as functional and sufficient: he is able to do the task and get back home – no meaningless wandering around the town.

From the point of view of managing responsibilities, the example shows how the participants jointly construct the client's preferred future and take the responsibility for meeting the recovery aims. Throughout the interaction, the client shows alignment to the premises of the support relationship and recovery aims (e.g. turns 8, 10, 12 and 14). The worker is taking the client to the community "out there". It is his responsibility to make it easier for the client to confront the community and to create a supportive relationship, as well as to strengthen the client to become a mobile citizen. In turn, the client recognises his responsibility to struggle with the barriers of active citizenship. There are techniques that he has to rehearse by himself. Going along is a vital working technique, as it enables workers to pave the way for the clients to the community. However, the technique has its limitations. It does not touch upon the root causes of the difficulties of being in the community. Nor does it allocate responsibilities to other community members. The critical issue is how the others encounter and involve vulnerable clients who try to (re)enter into the community.

Coaching: supporting a citizen to have strong willpower

The next example is from the same service as the previous one. The worker and the client are addressing essential restrictions in being able to go to the community during a home visit. For years the client has had such a poor physical and mental condition that it has been difficult for him to go out of the house. The intention of the interaction is to empower the client to become a mentally and physically stronger citizen.

Extract 4

1 WORKER: Yeah. But I think what you need to think about is where do you want to be in 12 months' time?
2 CLIENT: Well. It's like what I've just been saying in the kitchen. And I know. Don't get me wrong. I know I am one of these people where sometimes I'll say a lot of things and, you know …

3   WORKER: Put things off a bit.

4   CLIENT: I put things off, but I do need to motivate myself and start doing these things. And I think one thing that will help me more with outside. It's not because of people looking at me [unclear] but when I'm out there I think if I've got, like, a bit of weight knocked off me, it will improve my breathing.

5   WORKER: For your mobility as well.

6   CLIENT: Yeah. And I won't find that when I'm out I'm saying "Oh I need to go back in because blah, blah, blah". I feel as though I'd be able to stay out more.

7   WORKER: But there's got to come a point when you've got to say to yourself "Right. This is when it's going to change."

8   CLIENT: Yeah. I know.

9   WORKER: I mean, if you're serious enough about it, and I think you are.
      [The discussion continues by stating that the client's difficulties have lasted for ten years, and he will never get these years back or be able to change them.]

10   CLIENT: Exactly. So it's something that I need to do. But, I think, first things first. What I'm going to do, what I'm going to get sorted, and I am going to get it sorted as well ... I'm going to sort my house out, get it tidied, and I am going to get it tidied.

11   WORKER: Well. I mean, it's all part of like a new beginning, if you like.

12   CLIENT: Yeah. Get my house sorted out. But also I'm going to start going on the [exercise] bike. I'm going to start going on the [exercise] bike again and work at going on the bike. Because after a week of me going on the bike I do feel better. But I'm going to stick with it. And I am going to do it, and I'll let you know how I get on. I will tell you. I won't lie to you.

13   WORKER: No.

14   CLIENT: I'll tell you the truth. But I think if I just go on the bike a little bit and just feel that bit better in myself. I reckon I'll be more up for ...

15   WORKER: Yeah. You've got to look at the positive side. Just what benefits you'll gain from it.

16   CLIENT: So, yeah. I am going to do it. And I mean that as well. I'm not saying it and then like "Oh, I can't do it". My back does hurt me still. I do have problems with it, but it's not like it was when I had problems getting out of bed.

17   WORKER: Like you say, if you lost a bit of weight that probably ...

By posing a future-oriented question, the worker prompts the client to think about desirable and suitable future goals (turn 1). As a result, the client defines himself as a person who talks easily about things that need to be changed but cannot put the plans into practice (turns 2 and 4). In addition, the question prompts the client to produce a self-responsibilising account: "*but I do need to motivate myself and start doing these things*" (turn 4).

The worker shares the client's view that the current situation is undesirable, and there are things that need to be transformed and done. He calls for a life change and a turning point (turns 7 and 11). This championing for a life change triggers the client to respond by listing the things he has to do: "*Get my house sorted out. But also I'm going to start going on the [exercise] bike*" (turn 12). Interestingly, the client constructs a coach–client relationship and reaches out for the worker's support, but at the same time he looks to his own willpower: "*But I'm going to stick with it. And I am going to do it, and I'll let you know how I get on. I will tell you. I won't lie to you.*" (turn 12). The client categorises himself as a determined and honest citizen who is willing to try. He champions himself and talks against potential relapses (turn 16). The client starts to govern himself in a struggle for better well-being and health. He also recognises how being active itself gives self-confidence to become an even more active person (turn 14). The worker supports positive thinking and rational choice-making (turn 15).

The coaching technique seems to trigger the client to take responsibility: it is he who needs to start doing things. However, simultaneously the client asks for support and constructs the worker as a coach. It is the worker's responsibility to be there for the client and support him. Life change seems to require a person who follows, monitors and champions the "trying client". The example shows how strengthening the client's belief in himself is a crucial element in making an active citizen. Accordingly, at times mental health workers take the roles of life coaches and support the clients in the middle of their troubles, addictions and illnesses. Coaching is a useful working technique in many ways. It implies positive and empowering thinking. Clients are not left alone with their life projects. In addition, coaching is based on client choice, involvement and respect. Yet, coaching is very much an individualistic and self-responsibilising technique. Becoming an active citizen is interpreted as a personal project where a "non-active" citizen needs to be trained for the demands of everyday life and active membership of the community. Entering into the community seems to require being of a good enough fit. Coaching has the potential to give hope and the formation of new client categorisations, but what happens if the client fails the transformation task and sees him/herself as an even greater "loser" than before? What if the community does not welcome the client no matter how hard he/she tries to fit in? What then are the worker's responsibilities and possibilities? The risks of failure and defeat are always present in recovery processes.

Networking: gathering resources for the re-entering citizen

The last example[3] is from a Danish prison and probation service. The interaction takes place at a prison pre-release conference. Although a prison is a highly regulated environment, the early planning of inmates' re-entry into the community, supervision and community aftercare is a matter of great attention in today's policy and practice of probation (Petersilia 2003; Serin *et al.* 2010; Hardy 2014). The main purpose of the pre-release conference is to support the transition process from prison to the community by mobilising the networks around the client through a professional collaborative and coordinated effort. At the pre-release conference that is studied, there is a worker from the prison, the client (inmate), the client's mother and father, a worker from the job centre and a worker from the social services.

The client has been imprisoned several times in recent years and has been diagnosed with attention-deficit hyperactivity disorder (ADHD); his problems in everyday life due to the disorder are the main reason for organising the conference. At the time of the conference, the decision about whether and when the client would get his pre-release is yet to be made. The aim is therefore to plan the process of release and to justify the basis for such a decision. In addition, the conference is viewed as an important forum for securing inmates' access to social, health and housing services. The conference comprises an element of involuntariness for the client, although participation is not mandatory. If the client did not attend the conference, it would easily trigger client categories such as "not engaged", "non-active" and "not ready for re-entry to the community".

Extract 5

1   CLIENT: My name is [name] and it is me who is the project.
   [The other participants present themselves briefly.]

2   PRISON WORKER: We haven't set a timeframe [for the conference], because I didn't know how much each person has to contribute. We have many different things that we have talked about, anyway, that we would like to discuss at this conference. But now that there are so many of us, all with different approaches to [client's name], I will start by saying that the focus is on [client's name]. Around this table there are definitely a lot of people with lots of ambitions for [client's name]. And a lot of ideas of what's right, but we are not supposed to talk about that today. Today we'll talk about what it is [client's name] would like and how we can help him to do what he would like. This is what we need to try to focus on. I don't know if you would like to start [client's name], by telling us what you see as the most important thing that needs to be sorted out?

3   CLIENT: It is both my housing situation and then some support when I get out. To get some control of my everyday life again.

4   PRISON WORKER: Yes. And then we've talked about getting [client's name] finances sorted.

5   MOTHER: [client's name] is in Ribers [a national register of people with a poor credit history] and he has a very, very large debt.

6   PRISON WORKER: Yes. And also the financial support form, I think, so that you receive some money when you get out. It is you people from the municipality who should give us an idea of what the possibilities are for helping [client's name] financially and with something to do, a place to live and some support to make it all work.

7 JOB CENTRE WORKER: You have received housing assistance before, so you know a little about what kind of support we can offer from here? I remember when we talked before you went to prison, that you were interested in getting that back when you would be released again.

8 CLIENT: Yeah, and that it is under control, when I get released, so that it will not be two months after, as it then usually goes wrong.

[The discussion continues about the client's problems and specific needs of support. The client, the parents and the professionals talk about what would be the right solution and support for the client.]

9 SOCIAL SERVICE WORKER: But this has always been like that. What do you think yourself about what has to be done, so that it won't get out of control again?

10 CLIENT: It is, for example, if I have to attend to something I need someone to come by every morning. Just like here [in prison], where someone comes every morning to prick me with a stick to see if I am dead. Just to check up on if I am alive. Then the day is started. You are a little bit awake, and then you can get by yourself afterwards. It doesn't take a lot, but there has to be something or other.

With some irony, the client categorises himself, as the object of professional judgements and measures, as "the project" (turn 1). The prison worker resists this objectifying client category by emphasising that the focus of the conference is to clarify the client's wants and what the welfare workers can do to support his own objectives. Thus, the client is addressed in the conference interaction as an active participant, and the other members of the network are given responsibility to endorse his life project. The client acts as the expected "good" client, and expresses that he needs housing and support to *"get some control of my everyday life again"* (turn 3). His mother brings up an issue that makes it harder to manage the finance situation (turn 5). Following this, the prison worker interestingly addresses *"you people from the municipality"* and makes the welfare workers responsible for coming up with a solution for how to provide resources that the client needs for coping in the community (turn 6).

In turns 7 and 8, the risk is talked into being as the client presents himself as an individual who cannot necessarily manage himself without support that prevents him from getting things "wrong". Throughout the conference interaction, the welfare workers seek to involve the client and approach him as a collaborator to identify the preferred actions and outcomes concerning his re-entry into the community. In particular, the prison worker encourages the other welfare workers to acknowledge their joint responsibility for supporting the client in his attempts to lead a normal life on release.

Although the client seems to mainly act in the conference interaction according to the expectations of being an active participant, it can be seen in turns 8 and 10 that he sees a self-governing and independent citizenship as impossible (at least for now) for himself. In turn 9, the social service worker indicates that, for the client, things getting out of control is a long-term condition *"But this has always been like that*" (turn 9). She asks for the client's view on "*what has to be done*" (turn 9) so that an identified risk can be avoided. The client has a clear view on what helps him to be an active and participating citizen (and to avoid a negative trajectory of life in the community): "*I need someone to come by every morning*" (turn 10). The extract demonstrates how the client asks for support from the network in order to be able to participate in daily activities and to ensure independent living in the community.

In sum, the example illustrates the idea that to re-enter the community requires that both the client and the others take responsibility. The conference interaction may also be interpreted as being based on risk talk. The client, the welfare workers and the parents construct the pre-release situation as a (high) risk situation. The risk can be seen to be related to the essential but uncertain process of offender change; a transformation from being an active criminal (with a severe disorder) to a contributing, self-managing and responsible citizen (e.g. Rose 1996: 349; Serin *et al.* 2010: 55; Chapter 5 of this volume).

The networking technique (i.e. gathering resources and support) is conducted in an empowering way that encourages the client to express his wants and needs, and to use his experience-based expertise in preventing the risk of an unsuccessful release. Accordingly, the conference interaction can be seen to aim at strengthening the client's self-responsibility. However, the workers are identified also as being responsible for acting according to the client's wishes and for gathering resources for him, and, in this way, for working to prevent a negative future. Welfare workers become responsible subjects involved in, and bound to, the client's future.

Taking into consideration that the client has only scarce resources and is labelled in terms of stigma associated with the categories "ADHD" and "criminal", the shift from the prisoner to a free, recovered and self-governing actor is demanding. It can be assumed that the client recognises this and sets low expectations for himself in order to be able to manage everyday life without support and control. In this way, he resists the expectation of becoming a totally independent citizen. Therefore, the following questions can be asked: how should responsibilities be allocated between the client and the network? What is the client able to take responsibility for (despite his difficulties)? And, how would his responsibility best be realised? If one has a stigmatised life history and low societal status, and demanding present conditions, there are limited future choices and participation options. Despite this, the welfare workers and the client (though not the parents) are explicit in their interest in making the client an active and responsible citizen as part of the recovery and re-entry process. There are major complexities and obstacles in this transformation process.

Conclusion and discussion

The chapter has discussed the making of active citizens in the context of mental health and prison work. We have demonstrated how the clients struggle to be active in client–worker interaction and in their everyday life (see also Ponche *et al.* 2012).

Often there are concrete obstacles for the client (that are talked into being in client–worker interaction) in leaving their home and engaging with the neighbourhood. They struggle, for example, with a lack of energy, fears, anxiety, stress, stigma, poor mobility and health. The intent of the chapter has been to increase awareness of the issues tackled at the margins of welfare services by taking a look at the reality of the workers and the clients. In addition, we have identified working techniques (planning, questioning, going along, coaching and networking) used in promoting clients' participation and active citizenship in the community.

It can be argued following Dean (2002: 39) that governing by the active citizenship discourse "is quite compatible with a form of government of the state that places the question of order – whether personal or social – as its primary objective" (see also Ilcan and Basok 2004: 130–132). Within the discourse, order is constructed and obtained by privatising responsibility (Ilcan 2009) and setting norms for healthy, productive, social and undisruptive citizens. Furthermore, within the discourse, welfare workers and clients are approached as responsible subjects who ought to seek these attributes. Simultaneously, a line is drawn between those who manage to become active citizens and those who are not able or not willing to go through the required transformation process. Relevant questions (see also Fejes 2010) are:

- How does governance operate within the active citizenship discourse?
- What kinds of client categorisations are produced?
- Who are then addressed as being responsible for the recovery of citizens in the community?

It can be perceived from the analysis that making active citizens in the community is an interactional and complex achievement that requires negotiations concerning one's wants, needs, responsibilities, resources and risks. These negotiations comprise empowering and supportive as well as coercive potentials. Mental health work and prison work share a task to promote personal transformation and to ensure resources and networks for a better life in the community. Both the workers and the clients recognise their responsibilities in advancing successful re-entry and recovery processes. In particular, the clients account, explain and justify their endeavours to be active and self-responsible citizens (see Chapter 5).

Often the clients display themselves as active in their struggles to re-enter the community; but, according to cultural expectations of active citizenship (independence; workability; involvement in family life, civic society and voluntary work), the clients are nevertheless easily categorised as not being full citizens, i.e. having "conditional citizenship" (Hamer *et al.* 2014). In mental health and prison work, the accomplishment of active citizenship can be seen to form a continuum. There are many steps for the client to take: from being able to get out of one's home to being involved in self-help, leisure, family, study or work networks. Accordingly, active citizenship should be understood as a broad concept that comprises different levels of activities and participation. The clients' right to make choices about housing and services, as emphasised in consumerism and personalisation, is to be extended to the ways one chooses to be an active member of the community. Forced participation can be stressful and decrease one's well-being (Cummins and Lau 2003; Amado *et al.* 2013: 365). In order to be able to make active citizens in mental health and prison work in an ethical and constructive manner, it is crucial to ask people who have experienced marginalisation, illnesses and adversities what citizenship means to them, and in what way, if any, they hope for it to be strengthened (Rowe and Pelletier 2012: 379).

Active citizenship is a relational concept. Despite the individualistic aspects of active citizenship and the working techniques, full citizenship is made possible on the basis of a sense of community (Mezzina *et al.* 2006b: 72). Also, the root causes of "non-active" citizenship are profoundly social and structural in origin. The "loss of citizenship" is produced by complex factors such as isolation, stigmatisation, ill-health and devastating socioeconomic conditions (Mezzina *et al.* 2006a: 43). Welfare workers help vulnerable citizens living in the community to gain access to basic resources such as housing, income and support services. However, this does not ensure that vulnerable citizens have the status of a valued community member (Ponce *et al.* 2012: 361). Becoming a community member is a complex engagement process that is not planned, controlled or accomplished only by the state and welfare workers but also by ordinary co-citizens (Mezzina *et al.* 2006a: 59). This process is often replete with prejudices, stigmas, fears and moral expectations (e.g. Davidson *et al.* 2001; Hartwell 2004; Hamer *et al.* 2014: 208).

From mental health and prison work contexts, critical questions arise concerning the active citizenship discourse. Is active citizenship, after all, an unrealistic political ideal that excludes the majority of citizens? What is it to be sufficiently active and integrated in different contexts and in complex, devastating and stigmatising life situations (see Fakhoury and Priebe 2002; Turner 2012)? Re-entry into the community would be easier if the active citizenship discourse were "more self-reflecting on issues of cultural pluralism, the issue of difference, and the inclusion of a number of minorities in the definition of citizenship" (Bee and Pachi 2014: 108). Making active citizens is not a straightforward accomplishment, even if the participants share the intention to make the shift from "passive" to "active" client category. The shift is especially difficult if the socioeconomic situation (housing, income and support service) of the vulnerable citizens remains unsolved and unstable (see Jauffret-Roustide 2009: 169; Whiteford 2010). Thus, it is important in the future to obtain a balance between individualistic and collective working techniques and personal and social responsibilities, as well as to promote an inclusive community.

Notes

1 The example has been previously analysed from the point of view of clashing time discourses between the workers and the client in Juhila K., Günther, K. and Raitakari, S. (2015) "Negotiating mental health rehabilitation plans: Joint future talk and clashing time talk in professional client interaction", *Time & Society*, 24(1): 5–26.

2 The example has been previously analysed from the point of view of how integration is understood, discussed and promoted in the context of mental health home visits in Raitakari, S., Haahtela, R. and Juhila, K. (2015) "Tackling community integration in mental health home visit integration in Finland", *Health and Social Care in the Community*, DOI: 10.1111/hsc.12246.

3 Part of this example has been previously analysed from the point of view of service user identity negotiation in Berger, N.P. and Eskelinen, L. (2016) "Negotiation of user identity and responsibility at a prerelease conference", *Qualitative Social Work*, 15(1): 86–102.

References

Aharonson, E. and Ramsay, P. (2010) "Citizenship and criminalization in contemporary perspective: introduction", *New Criminal Law Review*, 13(2): 181–189.

Amado, A.N., Stancliffe, R.J., McCarron, M. and McCallion, P. (2013) "Social inclusion and community participation of individuals with intellectual/developmental disabilities", *Intellectual and Developmental Disabilities*, 51(5): 360–375.

Bee, C. and Pachi, D. (2014) "Active citizenship in the UK: assessing institutional political strategies and mechanisms of civic society", *Journal of Civic Society*, 10(1): 100–117.

Berger, N.P. and Eskelinen, L. (2016) "Negotiation of user identity and responsibility at a prerelease conference", *Qualitative Social Work*, 15(1): 86–102.

Bolzan, N. and Gale, F. (2002) "The citizenship of excluded groups: challenging the consumerist agenda", *Social Policy and Administration*, 36(4): 363–375.

Bosworth, M. (2007) "Creating the responsible prisoner: federal admission and orientation packs", *Punishment and Society*, 9(1): 67–85.

Cummins, R.A. and Lau, A.L.D. (2003) "Community integration or community exposure? A review and discussion in relation to people with an intellectual disability", *Journal of Applied Research in Intellectual Disabilities*, 16(2): 145–157.

Davidson, L., Haglund, K.E., Stayner, D.A., Rakfeldt, J., Chinman, M.J. and Kraemer, T.J. (2001) "'It was just realizing … that life isn't one big horror': a qualitative study of supported socialization", *Psychiatric Rehabilitation Journal*, 24(3): 275–292.

Davidson, L., Mezzina, R., Rowe, M. and Thompson, K. (2010) "'A Life in the Community': Italian mental health reform and recovery", *Journal of Mental Health*, 19(5): 436–443.

Dean, M. (2002) "Liberal government and authoritarianism", *Economy and Society*, 31(1): 37–61.

Eriksson, K. (2012) "Self-service society: participative politics and new forms of governance", *Public Administration*, 90(3): 685–698.

Fakhoury, W. and Priebe, S. (2002) "The process of deinstitutionalization: an international overview", *Current Opinion in Psychiatry*, 15(2): 187–192.

Fejes, A. (2010) "Discourses on employability: constituting the responsible citizen", *Studies in Continuing Education*, 32(2): 89–102.

Frazier, B.D., Sung, H.E., Gideon, L. and Alfaro, K.S. (2015) "The impact of prison deinstitutionalization on community treatment services", *Health & Justice*, 3(1): 1–12.

Garland, D. (2001) *The Culture of Control*, Chicago: University of Chicago Press.

Goddard, T. (2012) "Post-welfarist risk managers? Risk, crime prevention and the responsibilization of community-based organizations", *Theoretical Criminology*, 16(3): 347–363.

Hamer, H.P., Finlayson, M. and Warren, H. (2014) "Insiders or outsiders? Mental health service users' journeys towards full citizenship", *International Journal of Mental Health Nursing*, 23(3): 203–211.

Hardy, M. (2014) "Practitioner perspectives on risk: using governmentality to understand contemporary probation practice", *European Journal of Criminology*, 11(3): 303–318.

Hartwell, S. (2004) "Triple stigma: persons with mental illness and substance abuse problems in the criminal justice system", *Criminal Justice Policy Review*, 15(1): 84–99.

Hazleden, B. (2014) "Whose fault is it? Exoneration and allocation of personal responsibility in relationship manual", *Journal of Sociology*, 50(4): 422–436.

Ilcan, S. (2009) "Privatizing responsibility: public sector reform under neoliberal government", *Canadian Review of Sociology*, 46(3): 207–234.

Ilcan, S. and Basok, T. (2004) "Community government: voluntary agencies, social justice, and the responsibilization of citizens", *Citizenship Studies*, 8(2): 129–144.

Jauffret-Roustide, M. (2009) "Self-support for drug users in the context of harm reduction policy: a lay expertise defined by drug users' life skills and citizenship", *Health Sociology Review*, 18(2): 159–172.

Juhila, K., Günther, K. and Raitakari, S. (2015) "Negotiating mental health rehabilitation plans: joint future talk and clashing time talk in professional client interaction", *Time & Society*, 24(1): 5–26.

Kemshall, H. (2002) "Effective practice in probation: an example of 'advanced liberal' responsibilisation?", *The Howard Journal of Criminal Justice*, 41(1): 41–58.

Mezzina, R., Borg, M., Marin, I., Sells, D., Topor, A. and Davidson, L. (2006a) "From participation to citizenship: how to regain a role, a status, and a life in the process of recovery?", *American Journal of Psychiatric Rehabilitation*, 9(1): 39–61.

Mezzina, R., Davidson, L., Borg, M., Marin, I., Topor, A. and Sells, D. (2006b) "The social nature of recovery: discussion and implications for practice", *American Journal of Psychiatric Rehabilitation*, 9(1): 63–80.

Milbourne, L. (2009) "Valuing difference or securing compliance? Working to involve young people in community settings", *Children & Society*, 23(5): 347–363.

O'Malley, P. (2010) *Crime and Risk*, London: Sage.

Padfield, N. and Maruna, S. (2006) "The revolving door at the prison gate: exploring the dramatic increase in recalls to prison", *Criminology and Criminal Justice*, 6(3): 329–352.

Pathak, P. (2013) "From New Labour to New Conservatism: the changing dynamics of citizenship as self-government", *Citizenship Studies*, 17(1): 61–75.

Perron, A., Rudge, T. and Holmes, D. (2010) "Citizen minds, citizen bodies: the citizenship experience and the government of mentally ill persons", *Nursing Philosophy*, 11(2): 100–111.

Petersilia, J. (2003) *When Prisoners Come Home: Parole and prisoner reentry*, New York: Oxford University Press.

Pols, J. (2006) "Washing the citizen: washing, cleanliness and citizenship in mental health care", *Culture, Medicine and Psychiatry*, 30(1): 77–104.

Ponce, A.N., Clayton, A., Noia, J., Rowe, M. and O'Connell, M.J. (2012) "Making meaning of citizenship: mental illness, forensic involvement, and homelessness", *Journal of Forensic Psychology Practice*, 12(4): 349–365.

Priebe, S., Badesconyi, A., Fioritti, A., Hansson, L., Kilian, R., Torres-Gonzales, F., Turner, T. and Wiersma, D. (2005) "Reinstitutionalisation in mental health care: comparison of data on service provision from six European countries", *BMJ*, DOI: 10.1136/bmj.38296.611215.AE'.

Raitakari, S., Haahtela, R. and Juhila, K. (2015) "Tackling community integration in mental health home visit integration in Finland", *Health and Social Care in the Community*, DOI: 10.1111/hsc.12246.

Ramon, S. (2008) "Neoliberalism and its implications for mental health in the UK", *International Journal of Law and Psychiatry*, 31(2): 116–125.

Rose, N. (1990) *Governing the Soul: The Shaping of the Private Self*, Routledge: London.

Rose, N. (1996) "The death of the social? Re-figuring the territory of government", *Economy and society*, 25(3): 327–356.

Rose, N. (2000) "Government and control", *The British Journal of Criminology*, 40(2): 321–339.

Rose, N. (2002) "At risk of madness", in T. Baker and J. Simon (eds) *Embracing Risk: The changing culture of insurance and responsibility* (pp. 209–237), Chicago: University of Chicago Press.

Rowe, M. and Baranoski, M. (2011) "Citizenship, mental illness, and the criminal justice system", *International Journal of Law & Psychiatry*, 34(4): 303–308.

Rowe, M., Kloos, B., Chinman, M., Davidson, L. and Cross, A.B. (2001) "Homelessness, mental illness and citizenship", *Social Policy & Administration*, 35(1): 14–31.

Rowe, M. and Pelletier, J.-F. (2012) "Citizenship: a response to the marginalization of people with mental illness", *Journal of Forensic Psychology Practice*, 12(4): 366–381.

Sayce, L. (2000) *From Psychiatric Patient to Citizen: Overcoming discrimination and social exclusion*, Basingstoke, UK: Macmillan Press.

Sayce, L. (2003) "Beyond good intentions: making anti-discrimination strategies work", *Disability & Society*, 18(5): 625–642.

Schinkel, W. and van Houdt, F. (2010) "The double helix of cultural assimilationism and neo-liberalism: citizenship in contemporary governmentality", *British Journal of Sociology*, 61(4): 696–715.

Sells, D., Borg, M., Marin, I., Mezzina, R., Topor, A. and Davidson, L. (2006) "Arenas of recovery for people with severe mental illness", *Journal of Psychiatric Rehabilitation*, 9(1): 3–16.

Serin, R.C., Lloyd, C.D. and Hanby, L.J. (2010) "Enhancing offender re-entry: an integrated model for enhancing offender re-entry", *European Journal of Probation*, 2(2): 53–75.

Staeheli, L.A. (2013) "Whose responsibility is it? Obligation, citizenship and social welfare", *Antipode*, 45(3): 521–540.

Topor, A., Borg, M., Mezzina, R., Sells, D., Marin, I. and Davidson, L. (2006) "Others: the role of family, friends, and professionals in the recovery process", *American Journal of Psychiatric Rehabilitation*, 9(1): 17–37.

Turnbull, S. and Hannah-Moffat, K. (2009) "Under these conditions: gender, parole and the governance of reintegration", *The British Journal of Criminology*, 49(4): 532–551.

Turner, J. (2012) "Criminals with 'community spirit': practising citizenship in the hidden world of the prison", *Space & Polity*, 16(3): 321–334.

Uggen, C., Manza, J. and Thompson, M. (2006) "Citizenship, democracy, and the civic reintegration of criminal offenders", *Annals of the American Academy of Political and Social Science*, 605(1): 281–310.

Whiteford, M. (2010) "Hot tea, dry toast and the responsibilisation of homeless people", *Social Policy and Society*, 9(2): 193–205.

7 Negotiating risks, choices and progress in case-planning meetings

Christopher Hall, Lisa Morriss and Kirsi Juhila

Introduction

Much discussion has taken place in the human sciences regarding the increased concerns over the risks in social life under late modernity – an issue for both the citizen and the state. Citizens are increasingly expected to engage in behaviour that minimises their personal risk and allows them to anticipate potential dangers and thereby take more control of their lives (see Chapter 2). Similarly, the state aims to minimise risks by sometimes shifting responsibilities on to individuals and workers. A wide range of enabling programmes and "good life" advice have been developed to promote self-responsibility – in particular, attempting to identify, categorise and manage high-risk populations. As is discussed in Chapter 2, workers, who are charged with implementing government policies, are increasingly held accountable for preventing and managing the risks of their clients, and draw in particular on their relationship skills.

Risk and risk management clearly imply issues of responsibility. When assessing who is to blame for risks, attention turns to questions of who is responsible for managing them. As Giddens (1999: 8–9) comments: "Risks only exist when there are decisions to be taken.... The idea of responsibility also presumes decisions. What brings into play the notion of responsibility is that someone takes a decision having discernible consequences."

For those at the margins of the welfare state, allocating responsibility for making decisions regarding risks is a central concern. Citizens who are assessed as having serious problems in managing their lives responsibly are guided and controlled by various health, social and welfare workers in order to avoid unnecessary risks to themselves and society at large. Consequently, risks and choices become shared and negotiable issues between workers and clients; both parties have a responsibility to seek better risk assessments and make responsible choices. There is a wide variety of expert advice and opinions available to help individuals make "right and responsible" life decisions, and as Giddens (1991: 180) notes, "therapy should be understood and evaluated essentially as a methodology of life planning".

In this chapter, we demonstrate how risks and choices are negotiated in case-planning meetings dealing with substance abuse, mental health and housing problems. The focus is on how workers and clients assess progress and become more self-responsible when making choices and anticipating risks. Before considering the data, we ground our analysis in concepts of life planning and case management associated with the governmentality literature.

Life planning, risks and choices

Responsibilisation and the engagement of social and welfare workers with marginal groups centre around encouraging life planning and monitoring responsible choices by clients and workers. Drawing on Giddens, Ferguson (2001, 2003) has suggested that life planning is an appropriate frame to reformulate modern social work and social care, with its associations with "self-actualisation, healing and the acquisition of 'mastery'" (Ferguson 2001: 52). He writes that,

> [social] workers now routinely intervene into people's lives to assist them with their life-planning in the context of the new choices and problems they face. This may especially be at times of crisis when several options confront the service user who may be feeling overwhelmed by anxiety and the need to make decisions and be on the verge of or actually experiencing a "breakdown biography".
>
> (Ferguson 2001: 50)

By engaging with social work agencies, "individuals can also be seen as seeking to colonize the future for themselves as an intrinsic part of life planning" (Ferguson 2001: 51). Life planning should not thus be associated with only middle-class lifestyles:

> Giddens argues that the new life political agenda is perhaps even more relevant to the poor because the choices they face and the decisions they make with such limited resources are so consequential in terms of outcomes. Social work intervention in the context of life politics certainly has the scope to promote dependency and passivity and to be inappropriately constraining. Equally, though, it can permit engagement and re-appropriation of power by even the most marginalized service users.
>
> (Ferguson 2001: 49)

Later, however, Ferguson (2001: 51–52) suggests that only by cooperating with social services can service users make the most of the potential of the new life politics: "some 'involuntary clients' may never engage with the service". Ferguson thus sees the role of professionals as significant in clients' individual life planning: they can (re)produce clients' dependency (non-responsibility in one's own life) or they can support clients' empowerment and progress (and greater responsibility in one's own life). Ferguson's formulation of life planning resonates with recovery and resilience approaches; they position recovery as an individual responsibility (and a right) to master and change one's own life and resilience as a capability to transform oneself in the circumstances of many uncertainties (Coleman 1999; Welsh 2014: 20; Chapter 3 of this volume).

Governmentality and risk

The governmentality literature (discussed in Chapter 2) views the formulation of risk as not only an individual response to address the uncertainties of late modernity. Control of whole populations has been made possible in modern times by the development of expert knowledge to identify and categorise. Lupton (1999: 88–89) points this out as follows:

> For Foucault [in contrast to Beck and Giddens], however, expert knowledges are not transparently a means to engage in reflexivity. Rather they are seen as pivotal to governmentality, providing the guidelines and advice by which populations are surveyed, compared against norms, trained to conform with those norms and rendered productive.

Whereas Ferguson suggests that a social worker acts as an expert to support marginalised groups, the governmentality approach sees life planning technologies as primarily concerned with surveillance and controlling risks. Experts, like social and medical scientists, consultants and professional groups, construct categories for government – the unhealthy, the vulnerable, the dangerous and so on. As Lupton (1999: 89) says: "through these never-ceasing efforts, risk is problematised, rendered calculable and governable".

Government has developed a vast array of interventions, technologies and instruments: what Foucault (1991) terms as "the art of government". It is not merely the techniques and rationalities of government that are important, but also what Dean (1995: 560) calls the "axis of self-formation": "the ways in which particular domains of government have sought the cultivation and stylization of personal attributes and capacities, and marked out spaces for the supervised exercise of regulation of these capacities as arenas of freedom".

Government strategies, formulated in legislation, policies and practices, can be seen as persuasive and advisory but are also targeted at certain groups and may be coercive. Lupton (1999: 90–91) gives the example of how pregnant women are surrounded by and expected to engage with a vast array of advice, consultations, technological monitoring and lifestyle recommendations. Mostly, such interventions appear voluntary; however, it is the pregnant women's responsibility to engage with such interventions. Moreover, to "resist these strategies is difficult, for it is tantamount to declaring that the woman does not care about her own health and welfare and more importantly, that of the foetus she is carrying" (Lupton 1999: 92). Ignoring advice, missed appointments, or an inappropriate lifestyle can, in extreme cases, form the basis for professional concerns and potentially coercive interventions. In such a formulation, government takes place through a wide variety of everyday practices of agencies and workers rather than merely through legislation and policies. "The individualization of risks brings into question the very notion of social rights and is linked to a form of governing that seeks to govern not society but through the responsible and prudential choices and actions of individuals" (Dean 1999: 133).

Dean (1995, 1999) identifies case management as a particular form of risk rationality. Case management systems, developing from social work and clinical practice, have spread across practices in criminal justice, employment and education:

> Those judged "at risk" of being a danger to the wider community are subject to a range of therapeutic (e.g. counselling, self-help groups, support groups), sovereign (prisons, detention centres) and disciplinary (training and re-training) practices in an effort either to eliminate them completely from communal spaces (e.g. by various forms of confinement) or to lower the dangers posed by their risk of alcoholism, drug dependency, sexual diseases, criminal behaviour, long-term unemployment and welfare dependency.
>
> (Dean 1999: 143)

Case management has essentially been based on qualitative technologies – face-to-face diagnosis, professional judgement and case notes – but increasingly there are quantitative technologies in the form of risk assessments and practice instruments that are based on epidemiological calculations. Dean (1995) analyses policy and practices in youth unemployment in Australia, which aim to develop an "active system of income support" (Dean 1995: 568), which problematises the category of the long-term unemployed. The young person should be "job ready" and willing and able both to respond when a job is offered and to avoid "dependency on social security"; they are no longer a "claimant" but a "job seeker". At registration they are assessed as "job ready" or "at risk of long term unemployment" and allocated a case manager who "operates in what we can no doubt recognise, following Foucault, as a pastoral role, assessing the needs of clients, helping them prepare a plan to return to work and directing them towards the activities that enhance their job-readiness" (Dean 1995: 575).

Such activities are backed up with sanctions: failing an activity test, breaking an agreement or missing an appointment can result in lost allowances. As Dean (1995: 575) summarises:

> such pastoral activities amount to a kind of interface between governmental activities of the state (the provision of allowances and services etc.) and what might be thought of as a set of ascetic practices (self-examination, counselling, self-help groups, working oneself to improve one's job readi-ness, self-esteem, motivation levels, etc.).

Governmentality approaches identify the individual as taking on more respons-ibility for life planning, but less as a rational solution to late modernity and more as a self-governing, responsibilised citizen. The client of welfare services is encouraged to manage their own welfare and the associated risks, but only to the extent that such responsibilities and risks are in line with the legitimate practices and categories of government. Case management in particular is seen as a link between governmental ambitions to manage high-risk populations and technologies to construct active citizens and accountable workers.

Analysing everyday case management of risks and choices

The depiction of case management as a particular form of risk management technology is an important foundation for the analysis (Kemshall 2001: 98–99). Welfare work as empowering life politics is an optimistic, bottom-up approach that emphasises clients' individual life planning with the support of workers in an uncertain society, when the clients are faced with many choices. It puts faith in the ability of grass-roots level workers to strengthen clients' empowerment and recovery by providing advice in critical choice-making situations. Ferguson's (2001) suggestion to reformulate social work as life planning has unsurprisingly received a critical response (Garrett 2003, 2004; Houston 2004). Much of the argument has centred on the relative importance of structure and agency: how far can clients engage in self-actualisation and life planning when they are overwhelmed by inequality and oppression (Garrett 2003: 390)? And how much can workers help clients in this overwhelming situation? Are they also powerless? According to this criticism, individual life planning, in an empowering way, demands equally empowering societal, communal and organisational circumstances and resources.

In contrast to the life planning approach, a governmental approach tends to focus on the "top-down" mechanisms of surveillance and normalisation: the policies and procedures, the systems and the potential sanctions. Accordingly, it too has been criticised for being over-deterministic. Clarke (2006: 97) notes that "subjection is too often treated as a presumed effect in many analyses, rather than being treated as a problematic ambition which may or may not be achieved in practice". Rose *et al.* (2006: 100) accept that, to some extent, governmentality studies tend to concentrate on "the mind or texts of the programmer". Whilst the "iron cage" might be formidable, there are also opportunities for professional discretion and client resistance. McKee (2009: 474) concludes:

> By ignoring the messiness of realpolitiks, this top-down discursive approach neglects that subjection is neither a smooth nor a complete project; rather one inherently characterized by conflict, contestation and instability. Moreover, it downplays the way in which governmental programmes and strategies are themselves internally contradictory, continually changing and capable of mutation.

The related criticism of ignoring realpolitiks can be applied to the life politics approach in the sense that the ideal of supporting clients in their life planning in an empowering way can be confronted in many ways in the real practices of welfare work. So, in line with other chapters, we propose to examine in detail how responsibilities are managed in case-planning meetings. We concentrate on how risks and choices are negotiated, and how resistance may disrupt and undermine efforts to manage risk and choice. Since both the life politics and the governmental approaches include an idea of progress – in the sense of individual empowerment and recovery, or in the sense of becoming more self-responsible – we also analyse how progress is discussed and negotiated in the meetings.

Case management in community care

Case management approaches are applied in many welfare settings and client groups in need of health and social services, from older people to children being abused or neglected. Onyett (1998: 3) provides a simple definition: "Case management is a way of tailoring help to meet individual need through placing the responsibility for assessment and service coordination with one individual worker or team." He then provides the customary trajectory for professional interventions: assessment, planning, implementation, monitoring and review.

The cases and case management examined in this chapter are located in community mental health care settings. In addition to mental health, welfare work in these settings often also covers substance abuse and housing issues, as is the case in our case-planning exemplars. The adoption of case management in mental health marked a dramatic change in policy and practice. First, the move from the hospital to the community created a completely different environment for the client and hence a different relationship with the professional. Clients are no longer a captive audience as they are placed in a variety of living, recreational and work situations within normal communities. However, they may remain a risk to themselves and others.

Case management in mental health was developed in the USA in the 1970s, with multi-professional teams providing intensive support in the community (Floersch 2002: 42). Case managers regularly observe the details of the clients' lives and are involved in a wide range of mundane tasks concerning, in particular, employment, social skills, substance use, medication and housing (Floersch 2002: 50). As such, the case manager in mental health is involved in the close surveillance of those considered a risk. Case management in Europe has been developed more flexibly (Burns *et al.* 2001). In England, the Care Planning Approach (CPA) was introduced in 1990 (Department of Health 1990) and revised in 2008 (Department of Health 2008). The service is organised by joint health and social care Community Mental Health Teams, in which care coordinators (usually social workers, community psychiatric nurses or occupational therapists) develop the care plan and coordinate the contributions of other service providers (Simpson *et al.* 2003). In Finland, health and social care remain organisationally separate, without a keyworker coordinating all services for clients. However, joint case conferences do take place when it is considered necessary for particular clients and when tasks are allocated to both clients and workers.

Central to case management in community care is the case-planning meeting, where participants meet to coordinate the services for a client, assess the past, and plan forthcoming interventions in the client's service pathway and future life in general. The clearest example of case-planning meetings is the case conference or case review meeting. Previously a preserve of workers only, the case conference increasingly includes clients. Whilst there is research literature on the participation of clients (both parents and young people) in child welfare meetings (e.g. Hall and Slembrouck 2001; Hitzler and Messmer 2010), there is little written on meetings in adult services. Some interprofessional meetings take place without the client (Nikander 2003), which clearly changes the dynamics of the meeting (Hitzler and Messmer 2010).

There is, however, recent research on meetings in social security. Seing *et al.* (2012) examine meetings in Sweden which bring together professionals involved with people receiving sickness benefits to review their "work ability". As with CPA meetings, there is concern that the clients "take responsibility for the rehabilitation process". Seing *et al.* (2012: 557) note the centrality of the medical assessments and how the clients contribute little to the meetings, with health care staff acting as a "spokesperson" on their behalf. Wilińska and Bülow (2015) examine similar meetings with a focus on the emotions that are encouraged and resisted. Of particular relevance to the study of CPA meetings, the chair (from the Social Insurance Department) promotes the organisation's policy, in this case to encourage the client to be an active citizen, to return to work and to "feel good" about themselves (Wilińska and Bülow 2015: 2). Here also, timetables and the client's progress are features that are used as reference points to display the commitment by both workers and clients to the ambitions of the policy. Dall and Caswell (2015) examine rehabilitation meetings concerning appropriate training and benefits for clients. Although clients are present in the meetings, the analysis concentrates on the negotiations between the professionals. Such negotiations are concerned with the client making progress, and, as with Seing *et al.* (2012) above, there are occasions when the caseworker acts as a supporter of the client by questioning the relevance of the policy direction, which in this case is how far training promotes progress.

Oxley (2011) examines CPA meetings in England using turn-by-turn analysis. She concentrates on the way the client and the psychiatrist negotiate appropriate medication, which is a key feature of her data. In contrast to the responsibilisation orientation of our analysis, when it comes to medication, Oxley (2011: 65) finds that professionals were reluctant to concur with the clients' requests to reduce dosage, which could be seen as a sign of progress: "thus references by professionals to dose seem to work to quantify and professionalise, rather than open up conversation about the service user's experiences and preferences of medication".

Progress was, however, encouraged when discussing work and leisure activities, with the client taking responsibility for promoting the benefits of work. As a psychiatrist inquires: "you're hoping to progress on from there (voluntary work)" (Oxley 2011: 70). Even so, Oxley (2011: 90) concludes that the discourses of illness collide with progress in employment if they risk worsening the client's mental health. In summary, case-planning meetings in various settings draw on policies to promote the progress of the client and the management of responsibilities.

Risks, choices and progress in case-planning meetings

Two case-planning meetings

In the following analysis of two case-planning meetings, we first show how the analysis of talk and interaction can provide understanding of categories and identities. What versions of people do the participants appear to construct, act out and negotiate during meetings, both in regard to themselves and to others? Second, we pay attention to how workers give advice and persuade clients to make non-risky choices and how these choices relate to progress in clients' lives. Our third interest is to examine clients' responses and possible resistance towards advice. The two planning meetings are located differently within the case-planning process: the first reviews the client's progress in a particular supported housing project, whereas the second is a multi-professional meeting that reviews all aspects of the client's life. In both meetings, the client is mostly the principal addressee; this is in contrast to other meetings where the professionals address one another with the client as a "bystander" (Hall and Slembrouck 2001; Seing *et al.* 2011).

Making non-risky choices means progress (or risk choices mean regression)

The first planning meeting[1] is at a Finnish supported housing and floating support service run by a non-governmental organisation. The unit offers a community-based alternative to hospital or nursing homes for people of working age who suffer from both mental health and substance abuse problems. It is not meant to be a permanent placement; instead, the principal aim of this intervention is to strengthen the clients' ability to lead normal and independent lives. After spending a reasonable amount of time in the service, the clients are expected to integrate into society as more self-responsible citizens. The ideal pathways are seen as linear and progressive. The professional tool in creating these pathways is a rehabilitation plan. Making the plans and reviewing them on a regular basis is an inherent part of the service's practices. The plans include the aims of individual recovery, assessment of progress and possible setbacks, and the mapping of all services that are involved or needed in rehabilitation processes. In practice, plans are processed in a planning meeting where a client and his/her keyworkers are present.

In the following meeting, two keyworkers and a client discuss the client's rehabilitation prospects. The workers display their concern about the client's current situation: the aims written in the original plan have not been fulfilled. The client in question is a woman in her early twenties, living alone. She has been diagnosed as having Asperger's syndrome, ADHD (attention deficit hyperactivity disorder) and a substance abuse dependency that is in an acute phase at the time of the meeting. The meeting is very short (18 minutes). It begins with a summary of the client's current situation presented by the worker.

Extract 1.1

1   WORKER 1: So the situation is this, [Client], that each and every application for education you've made has bounced back, and that's because of your continuous drinking, and the latest reply was from the rehabilitation centre: the psychologist in the education committee phoned to say that they won't accept your application because of your use of alcohol. In the same way, your application for trial work was rejected because of your drinking. And we've now come to a point where something must be done. I mean, you are no longer in control of things and your liver will soon go "pop".

The summary draws a pessimistic picture of the client's situation. The worker produces evidence for this critical assessment by listing unsuccessful service contacts and applications from the client's near past: all education applications have been rejected, as well as the application for trial work. Lack of success is explained by causal accounting (Bull and Shaw 1992; Raitakari *et al.* 2013; Chapter 5 of this volume): the client's continuous alcohol use is presented as the real reason for the current situation. The reported speech by the psychologist supports this conclusion (Wooffitt 1992; Holt 1996: 225–226; Juhila *et al.* 2014: 156–159). The listed past failures, rejected applications for education and trial work due to drinking, give grounds for the assessment that the client's future will probably not be any better; the direction could become even more regressive. The way in which the keyworker summarises the current situation makes it clear that this is not what the keyworkers and the client have agreed earlier when formulating the rehabilitation plan. She categorises the client as a person *"no longer in control of things"*. In other words, the client is constructed as not having enough self-responsibility for transforming the regressive direction in her life to a progressive one. The worker identifies the client's continuous drinking as a major future risk for both the client's future employability and health (*"your liver will soon go 'pop'"*). So, she defines this moment as a last chance to change the direction: *"we've now come to a point where something must be done"*. The summary has a blaming tone (*"your drinking"*, *"your use of alcohol"*), but on the other hand, positioning the client as having no control (cf. alcoholism as a disease) also hints that the client has an excuse for her behaviour. Furthermore, using *"we"* refers to the client's and the worker's shared responsibility for solving the situation. The worker appears to give advice for both the client and herself that something should be done immediately to prevent a future catastrophe. The client responds to the worker's opening turn and summary by displaying concern about her health.

Extract 1.2

2   CLIENT: I actually meant to ask you, so with the hepatitis, I may get cirrhosis of the liver.

3   WORKER 1: Well, you may get it faster than you normally would.
4   CLIENT: You mean I could already have it now?
5   WORKER 1: Well, I couldn't say about that, but it's not going to help you at all here if you don't recognise that you have an alcohol problem.
[discussion about the situation and the possibility of the cirrhosis continues for a while.]

The client treats the worker as a medical expert (although she is not a doctor) by asking her whether she is in danger of developing cirrhosis of the liver, since she already has hepatitis. In response, the worker does not allay the client's concern, as she estimates that the client is at risk of developing the disease faster than normal. The increasing concern, almost panic, is present in the client's next question: "*You mean I could already have it now?*" However, hearing the client's concern, the worker does not reassure the client nor refer her to a doctor but instead displays uncertainty (she could not say whether the client already has the disease). She then emphasises the client's agency and responsibility; for a start, she has to recognise she has an alcohol problem. The client does not directly resist this category option (being an alcoholic), although she does not accept it either. Instead, she continues "worry talk" of the possibility of the risk of cirrhosis. So, the worker and the client seem to be on different tracks in the interaction; the client is first of all concerned about her health condition (medical category) whilst the worker is more concerned about the client's life prospects in general if the drinking continues and the client does not recognise that it is a problem (social category). Shortly after this exchange, the worker closes the disease talk by presenting two optional future choices for the client's life and correspondingly for the rehabilitation work with her.

Extract 1.3

22   WORKER 2: And we've got two options here, so you'll know, you'll understand what we're dealing with. We're dealing with a very serious and problematic disease, with alcoholism, and what worries us here is that you're so very young, you've got your future ahead of you and that we should find a future career for you. And indeed, no college will accept you if you don't do something about the problem yourself. And you can't think, the way your friends say, that you'll be financed by the social services to the end of your life. You're stuck with institutions; you'll be in and out of the mental hospital the rest of your days. From the institution to community care, from community care to rehabilitation, institution, health centre, until you die. This is the truth. What we need now is treat—
23   CLIENT: But what I've said to my friends, that the way I live, I tell them that this is just temporary.
24   WORKER 2: Yes, but the way you're going about it, it's going to be permanent.

Two options are described as extremes between which the client is expected to make a choice. The first, and preferred, option is that the client herself starts addressing the main problem of alcoholism and becomes a recovery-oriented person. The alternative, "wrong", option is to continue in the same way. Although the worker defines alcoholism as a serious disease, she argues that getting rid of it is a matter of choice and conscious decision. So, she combines medical and social categories in assessing the situation. The risks of choosing the wrong option are constructed as fatal: endless revolving in marginal social services and a gradual regression. The worker thus strongly advises the client to choose the non-risky, "do something about the problem" option. The client responds to these future visions, and the advice to choose the preferred option, by claiming that her current way of living is temporary; it will probably change in the future, but a decision to change it right now is not perhaps necessary. Talk about the temporary situation seems to refer to the client's age; the client categorises herself as a young person in transition, whose life will steady in the future. The other keyworker disagrees with this interpretation and categorisation: there is a clear risk that the temporary situation will turn into a permanent, lifelong way of living.

What is at stake is a particular categorisation of a client who recognises that she has an alcohol problem (Seing *et al.* 2012: 554). If she accepts this identity, the client is treated in this meeting as capable of directing her life and making a right, responsible choice in a tricky situation. To support the preferred option, the workers spell out clearly for the client the serious consequences of the wrong, risky choice, as well as the better future vision related to the right choice. The message is that from this point on, it is up to the client to choose which path to follow. The client formulates a different life plan for herself, as she appears reluctant to accept the workers' categorisation, and instead sees her situation as being temporary and one that she can bring to an end. Both parties then formulate the future life plan for the client to determine, although the prospects are defined differently. This conversation is thus an example of client responsibilisation in two senses. At the end of the planning meeting, the workers strongly persuade the client to take a next step based on their future prospect and related life plan by "changing her attitude" and by accepting a referral to substance abuse treatment. The client hesitantly accepts this plan and the associated identity as a person having an alcohol problem.

Making non-risky choices means non-progress

We will now examine extracts from an English CPA meeting to assess how the risks are managed, and how the life planning work is negotiated and contested by workers and clients. As mentioned above, being managed through the CPA system, the client has a named care coordinator and an initial comprehensive multi-disciplinary, multi-agency assessment to formulate a care plan which is then reviewed at least once a year (usually more often) at a formal multi-disciplinary, multi-agency CPA review meeting. The Guidance (Department of

Health 2008: 7) includes a *Statement of Values and Principles*, stating that this approach to individuals' care and support "puts them at the centre and promotes social inclusion and recovery". However, Gould (2013) found that CPA care plans predominantly emphasise clinical outcomes, medication and risk; indeed, the meeting discussed below includes talk about risk and crisis planning in order to meet the requirements of the CPA review form. For example, the psychiatrist attempts to close the meeting before risk has been discussed, but is prevented by doing so by the chair of the meeting.

PSYCHIATRIST: I think unfortunately we have to stop it there. I'm expecting to have a patient waiting outside whose appointment —
CHAIR: Just another minute, can we just discuss risk at the minute?

Our contention is that life planning is carefully managed in the meeting by celebrating instances of progress and displaying choice, whilst managing instances that might be seen as risk, regression or resistance.

This is a meeting to review the care plan of a middle-aged woman with a long history of mental illness, who is living in a supported housing unit. The meeting is chaired by the team manager, as the social worker is off sick. Others present are the client, the housing support worker, the support worker from the Community Mental Health Team and the psychiatrist (who does not speak during the extract). In the extracts, the following symbols are used:

- (2) = pauses in seconds
- (.) = pauses under a second
- °talk° = silent voice
- <I like you> = talk is slowing down.

Extract 2.1

1 CHAIR: We talked about your housing. You're happy to stay at [supported housing] at the moment? Yeah?
2 CLIENT Hmm.
3 CHAIR Yeah. [To the housing support worker] Anything for you there about that?
4 HOUSING SUPPORT WORKER: Erm, what's happening at the moment, [Chair], is, you know, it's a two-year period ...
5 CHAIR: Yes.
6 HOUSING SUPPORT WORKER: ... at [supported housing], and we can always ask for an extension.
7 CHAIR: Yes.
8 HOUSING SUPPORT WORKER: And even though [Client] has this big massive package of support in, it's kind of been identified with [Social Worker] and [Client] and myself.

9   CHAIR: Mm.

10   HOUSING SUPPORT WORKER: It's (2) still not quite enough in the evening.

11   CHAIR: OK.

12   HOUSING SUPPORT WORKER: And we actually went to look at [a residential unit], erm, on (.).

13   CLIENT: Tuesday.

14   HOUSING SUPPORT WORKER: Tuesday, [Client].

15   CHAIR: Right.

16   HOUSING SUPPORT WORKER: And would you like to say (.), erm (.), talk about [a residential unit] and what it was like and what you've decided and (.) what's happening?

17   CLIENT: Well, I like it.

18   CHAIR: Do you?

19   CLIENT: It's nice.

20   CHAIR: It is a lovely place, yeah. And it is the evenings isn't it, that's your little ...

21   CLIENT: Yeah.

22   CHAIR: ... area of concern, isn't it. Because you get a bit lonely and isolated and call the crisis team a lot. So, [residential unit], there's 24-hour staffing isn't there, there? So you're making a positive decision, are you, to perhaps move there?

23   CLIENT: Hmm.

24   CHAIR: Yeah. Okay. Are you perhaps going to visit again just to make sure you've made the right choice?

25   CLIENT: Yeah, I'm going on Tuesday for my dinner.

26   CHAIR: Are you? OK, OK, that's good. You'll probably know a few people there, I suspect, once you go there a few times. Yeah, OK, so that's good that we had that little reminder that you might be moving on. OK, about your finances then, you manage your money, well, you pay your bills. Do you know what benefits you actually get?

[The chair asks if this client has been affected by recent changes in benefits.]

The chair has been covering the questions in the CPA form. She introduces the topic of housing and asks the client whether she is happy to stay in the current supported housing, to which the client agrees (turns 1 and 2). The housing support worker is invited to comment and produces a different future for the client. She does not immediately challenge the preferred formulation established by the chair, but produces a story that enlists the chair's agreement on key preliminaries, which is an example of recipient design (Sacks *et al.* 1974). A story preface seeks an extended turn: *"what's happening at the moment, [Chair]"* (turn 4). A contrast is provided between the ideal pathway – the unit is time limited although an extension could be sought – and an unpreferred alternative one: the client is receiving extra support, using upgraded terms *"big massive support"* (cf. Wilińska and Bülow 2015).

Consequently, the social worker, the client and the housing support worker all agree that it is not working. The housing support worker is careful to play down her agency in each of these steps, and gets an approving response from the chair after each non-controversial statement (turns 5, 7, 9 and 11). However, the extent of the apparent problem is delicate but specific – *"not quite enough in the evening"* (turn 10) – and depicts a low level of failure but also reminds the chair of the absence of staff at the unit in the evening: it is untenable to continue the current placement. Note the pause in turn 10 before stating the problem.

The strong *"OK"* affiliation in turn 11 by the chair enables the housing support worker to describe the actions to further the alternative pathway: namely a visit had been made to a residential home, which is the opposite of the notion of progress. The client's voice is strongly involved, first to complete the housing support worker's turn 13 and then to encourage a positive opinion – *"I like it"* (turn 17). The latter is set up and responded to as the client's choice in several senses: *"what it was like"* (client description), *"what you've decided"* (client choice) and *"what's happening"* (subsequent action) (turn 16). Such a formulation facilitates strong displays of affiliation between the chair and the client (turns 17–21). In turns 20 and 22, the chair picks on the problem of the evenings by encouraging alignment from the client – *"yeah"* (turn 21) – but also highlights the inappropriate demands on the crisis team (turn 22) and thereby aligns with the housing support worker's concern. Clients in supported housing should not call the crisis team too often. The chair asks if the client has made a decision, although this is hedged with *"perhaps move there"* (turn 22) and *"visit again"* (turn 24). By offering advice to visit again, the chair appears to suggest that options are still open but then closes the topic in a positive acknowledgement – *"OK, OK that's good"* (turn 26).

The comment in turn 26 – *"so that's good that we had that little reminder that you might be moving on"* – suggests the chair is displaying a mild criticism that a major change in an unpreferred direction has been presented to the meeting as a *fait accompli*. The term *"a little reminder"* is ironic as it is not "little" and "reminder" implies actions taken elsewhere and now reported to the meeting as an established state of affairs. The housing support worker's indirectness in introducing the decision has spared her possible criticism. This exchange is co-constructed storytelling with elements of story structure identified by Labov (1972). Whilst there is no coda, there is an orientation – *"what's happening at the moment"* (turn 4), a complication – *"it's not quite enough"* (turn 10) and a resolution, an alternative pathway and an evaluation – *"that's good"* (turn 26). The co-constructed aspect is especially prominent, with the housing support worker and client sharing the telling of the resolution, and the chair and client sharing the evaluation.

At this stage of the meeting, the client is categorised as inappropriately placed in supported housing and as not ready for rehabilitation, despite having made progress in areas already discussed. She is also supported to make positive and appropriate choices. The exchange displays three overlapping formulations – client choice, professional risk assessments, and ideologies of progress and recovery. It is suggested that a combination of professional risk assessment and client choice is required to justify a suspension of the progress/recovery (Dall and Caswell 2015). As with Oxley (2011: 76), concerns about risk put progress on hold.

A few minutes later, another change that affects the client's independence is introduced.

Extract 2.2

39. HOUSING SUPPORT WORKER: And [Social Worker] in the process, she's either completed it or in the process of completing it.
40. SUPPORT WORKER: And also [Chair], [Social Worker] and [Client] have both agreed that (.) [Client] may be put on appointeeship.
41. HOUSING SUPPORT WORKER: °Yeah°.
42. SUPPORT WORKER: But just due to her managing skills, her managing her money.
43. CHAIR: Well, that sounds a bit contradictory, to be honest.
44. SUPPORT WORKER: It does, but—
45. HOUSING SUPPORT WORKER: It's, it's been … it's, it's, it's not about paying the bills and everything. It's just, at the minute, there's a friendship – am I OK to speak about this, [Client]?
46. CLIENT: Hmm.
47. HOUSING SUPPORT WORKER: There's a friendship, but it's at the cost of [Client] financially, but it hasn't been seen as financial abuse. I think [Social Worker] may have spoken to you about it, and it was agreed that appointeeship … to speak to [Client] that [Client] agreed to it, and that was going ahead. And it's just that this person is a friend, but she kind of goes on a bit at [Client], and [Client] ends up buying her things or paying for things.
48. CHAIR: Right, OK. Do you feel pressured?
49. CLIENT: Hmm.
50. CHAIR: And do you feel you can't say no?
51. CLIENT: Yeah.
52. CHAIR: OK, all right, because on the one hand you've got very good evidence that you can manage your money, daily bills etc. So in terms of the local authority taking responsibility for your money, and then you then being given money on a regular basis and having your bills paid, it takes away a bit of your independence, really.
53. CLIENT: Hmm.
54. CHAIR: And you've actually got quite a lot of capacity to understand your money apart from this one area.
55. HOUSING SUPPORT WORKER: Well, what's happened on occasions is that [Client]'s been left without money.
56. CHAIR: Oh, has she?
57. HOUSING SUPPORT WORKER: And not even money for her phone and we've had to get a food parcel.

58. CHAIR: OK, OK.
59. HOUSING SUPPORT WORKER: But she still pays her bills.
60. CHAIR: Right, OK.
[Chair suggests a different way of managing the client's money]

After a report from the housing support worker that the client is able to pay her bills on time, the support worker reports that it has been decided to arrange for her money to be managed by the local authority through an appointeeship. This is one of the few occasions that the support worker speaks in the meeting, and the housing support worker's soft "°*Yeah*°" (turn 41) can be heard as indicating that she has omitted reporting this development. The chair reacts with some indignation, "*Well, that sounds a bit contradictory, to be honest*" (turn 43). The support worker struggles to provide an explanation, and when the housing support worker takes over she also finds it hard to begin "*it's, it's been (.) it's, it's, it's not*" (turn 45). In contrast to the housing support worker's story about the visit to the residential home in Extract 2.1, here there is no preliminary pre-paratory story or involvement of the client in the explanation.

The housing support worker begins to construct a further refinement in the client's characterisation: she can manage bills, but there is a problem with a friend who is taking advantage of her. The housing support worker again develops a story, and this time looks to the client for permission for an extended turn – "*am I ok to speak about this, [Client]*" (turn 45). The housing support worker's story starts with a number of attempts to categorise the problems: a "*friendship*" that is "*at the cost of [Client] financially*" but which is not "*financial abuse*" (turn 47). An agreement had been made that appointeeship is appropriate, and the chair herself may have been consulted. The client has also agreed. Again a process is going ahead which is the opposite of progress. Now the housing support worker provides the story behind the decision: the problem is a friend who somehow persuades the client to spend money on her. In contrast to the previous story, the explanation here provides a resolution first – seek appointeeship, and only then is the complication introduced – spending money on a friend.

Also unlike the previous extract, the housing support worker has not involved the client in the telling and has spoken about her predominantly in the third person, thus indicating that this is essentially professional talk. This is in contrast to a "we" formulation in collaboration with the client, noted by Dall and Caswell (2015). The chair switches back to client–professional talk and asks the client if she feels under pressure (turn 48). She now puts her dilemma to the client: you are good with paying bills, and the appointeeship will take away some independence. The housing support worker interrupts the dialogue and reports the serious incident (turn 55); the chair appears to accept this (turns 58 and 60) and changes the topic.

In this extract we have seen a further refining of the client's characterisation: she is capable of independence on money matters, but at the same time she is vulnerable in other aspects. The assessment of risk has again challenged her progress towards further independence. Here, however, the chair has turned to the client to question the decision to progress with the appointeeship. In the following discussions, the chair suggests an alternative to protecting the client's money which could be pursued.

Extract 2.3

70   CHAIR: Do you understand what that means in terms of the local authority managing your money?
71   CLIENT: (3) Erm (3), I think so.
72   CHAIR: I think we probably need to go over that a bit more really. Yeah. It's your money (1) then you just get support to manage it, OK? If you wish to take it out then you take it out, OK, but you're just encouraged to perhaps budget a little bit more closely really.
73   CLIENT: Yeah.
74   CHAIR: They will actually pay all your bills for you, but that would be taking away a bit of your independence.
75   HOUSING SUPPORT WORKER: [indistinct]
76   CHAIR: So I think you should put in the plan that it helps you to do what you can do.
77   HOUSING SUPPORT WORKER: Yeah.
78   CHAIR: Really, I think [Social Worker] should talk to her a bit more about that.
79   SUPPORT WORKER: Yeah. You've been on appointeeship before, haven't you, [Client]?
80   HOUSING SUPPORT WORKER: Yeah.
81   CHAIR: Oh, so you do, you're fully aware then.
82   HOUSING SUPPORT WORKER: Yeah, and then when we had the meeting, [Social Worker] did go through the appointeeship and what it meant and that's when [Client] agreed to it.
83   CHAIR: Yeah.
84   HOUSING SUPPORT WORKER: So it has been discussed in depth.
85   CHAIR: OK, OK, erm … Are you aware that once you go to [residential unit] your finances will be affected?
86   CLIENT: (4) It'll be?
87   CHAIR: Your money <will (.) come down (.) if you do take (.) the place> at this residential care.
88   CLIENT: How much will I get, then?
89   CHAIR: Well, have you ever been detained under the Mental Health Act under Section 3 at all? I don't think you have.
90   CLIENT: No.
91   CHAIR: No, if you had you'd have been entitled to what's called 117 after-care, where your finances would be – the cost for the residential care would be paid for by the local authority, but you will have a contribution to make to that. And so that will mean that you'll be left, after all the deductions, with around about £20, £22 a week. And then you'll get

the mobility element of DLA, but the care element will be suspended whilst ever you're in residential care, because that goes towards the care, basically. So you do need to seriously think about all of this, OK?

92 HOUSING SUPPORT WORKER: Yeah. We have spoken about doing a break-down, haven't we [Client], because we weren't sure how financially [Client] was going to be affected, but once we've found out the cost we were going to do a breakdown, weren't we?

93 CHAIR: Hmm.

94 HOUSING SUPPORT WORKER: Because it was something on that basis whether you were going to decide yes or no.

95 CHAIR: Yeah. You need to be fully clear about what money you'd be left with, OK? Obviously you won't be paying bills, and you won't be paying for food, and you won't be paying for cleaning or anything like that. So the money that you have is pocket money, basically, yeah OK, but you need to think about that, all right?

96 CLIENT: Hmm.

97 CHAIR: OK. I don't think I've missed any areas. Let's just look at the level of risk now, OK? Today, how safe do you feel in yourself?

The chair now asks the client if she understands what it means to have her money managed by the local authority. The client's hesitancy at turn 71 prompts the chair to suggest that it needs to be discussed further. She makes a contrast between the client having access to her money and the local authority acting on her behalf, and contends that this will take away some of the client's independence. At turn 75, the housing support worker appears to seek the floor [indistinct]. In turns 76 to 78, the chair continues to talk to the client but also acknowledges the housing support worker as an addressee. The instruction to "*put in the plan*" is directed at the housing support worker, whereas in the comment "*helps you to do what you can do*", the "*you*" refers to the client. The support worker and the housing support worker now provide two reasons why the appointeeship is not a problem. First, the support worker points out that the client has had it in the past, addressing the client (turn 79). Second, the housing support worker reports that it was discussed at the meeting, and concludes that it "*has been discussed in depth*" (turn 84), which is a strong counter to the chair's suggestion that there should be further discussion.

Whilst the chair accepts at turn 81 that the client might be "*fully aware*" of the implications of the appointeeship, at turn 85 she uses the issue of the client's loss of control of her money to question the placement in residential care. Again the client now appears less certain (turns 86 and 88). The problem is presented now as "*your money will come down*" in residential care (turn 87). Note the short pauses in this explanation by the chair in turn 87, and the general slowing down in the talk. Freese and Maynard (1998: 204) note that speech tends to slow down when delivering bad news in everyday conversation.

The chair spends some time explaining the complexities of payments to answer the client's question "*how much will I get, then?*" (turn 88). The description mentions legislation, contributions and deductions but then mentions a figure of £20–£22 per week plus part of another benefit (DLA or disability living allowance) (turn 91). Unlike the previous exchange, the chair does not check with the client to see if she has understood the explanation. The final statement in the turn, "*so you do need to seriously think about all of this*" (turn 91), does not invite any clarification, but, as in Extract 2.1, the chair advises the client to re-think this option. Instead, the housing support worker takes the next turn and locates the solution in a proposal "*to do a breakdown*" of the client's money by involving the client in this plan. The housing support worker now indicates that the proposed move is still to be decided – "*whether you were going to decide yes or no*" (turn 94). The chair can now suggest that the client re-evaluate the proposed move in financial terms (turn 95).

Therefore, in this meeting, the client appears not to conform to a linear notion of progress which might be expected to be the focus of a CPA meeting. As with the analysis of the previous meeting, it is the categorisation of the client that is disputed, only here the disagreement is between the workers (Seing *et al.* 2012). The categorisation of the client proposed by the social worker and the housing support worker is ambiguous – she has made progress towards independence but is also at such risk that a placement with less independence is being proposed. The chair considered this "*contradictory*" (turn 43) as it would reduce the client's independence and is the opposite of progress. Decisions have been made by the client, the social worker and the housing support worker prior to the meeting. The chair, however, directs the workers and the client to reconsider both decisions, by displaying the client's lack of understanding and in particular her concern about having less money. She uses advice-giving to the client as a way of undermining the workers' explanations of the problem. It is suggested that participants in the meeting draw on three forms of talk to characterise the client and establish formulations of action – progress, risk and choice. All three provide legitimate arguments and are available to formulate preferred categories of the client and undermine others.

Conclusion and discussion

In reviewing the literature, it was suggested that life planning, case management and recovery practices can be seen as empowering vulnerable citizens to make critical decisions and responsible choices in much the same way as all citizens aim to manage risks in late modernity. Alternatively, such practices can be seen as technologies of government to control and keep under surveillance those whose lifestyles challenge conventional expectations and make demands for what are considered to be excessive state support and dependency. As with other chapters in this book, we have demonstrated that in everyday encounters between workers and clients at the margins of welfare services, characteristics of interactions include structure and practice, constraint and discretion, and negotiation and resistance.

Case management and care planning are clearly systems of surveillance and monitoring, which establish measurable and reportable expectations of conduct within arenas of oversight for both clients and workers. As mentioned earlier, Dean (1995: 575) notes that case management contains a particularly strong configuration of sanctions and ascetic practices; not just control but also personal examination. When driven by notions of progress that require movement towards reduced dependency and greater independence, all parties are locked into a system of timetables and bureaucratic oversight. However, inevitably there are gaps and inconsistencies when policies and procedures are faced with the complexities of the needs of vulnerable clients and scarce resources. Workers and clients must conform to progress and recovery and make responsible decisions, but risks must also be managed and anticipated.

Case-planning meetings in particular are occasions on which the exigencies of peoples' lives are formulated in terms of principles of progress, risk and choice, thereby promoting policy (Dall and Caswell 2015). Seing *et al.* (2012: 555) describe meetings as having a supportive and controlling function to promote the policy but also to fit the client into that policy. In both the meetings examined, the concern is with a candidate negative categorisation of the client and with the present state of affairs formulated as untenable. In the first meeting, the client is not achieving the progress in work and education that was expected, and is seen as being in danger of becoming an alcoholic, with both medical and social consequences. In the second meeting, despite managing well in some areas (e.g. paying her bills), the client is considered too vulnerable (isolated and lonely) for her present placement, as she constantly calls the crisis team and has been taken advantage of by a friend.

In both cases, progress is not going well and the risks are high. However, the allocation of responsibility to address these risks is managed differently. In the first meeting, it is considered that the client needs to take on the dangers of her alcohol abuse herself: both the present manifestations and future possibilities. She needs to address her self-identity. The client resists such a formulation, seeing it as a temporary situation which she can change. Both the workers and the client allocate her responsibility for her situation and future progress, even if the workers consider that she is making the wrong choices. In the second meeting, there are different versions of the client being proposed by the workers. The service providers suggest a more dependent status for the client, who should move to a more restrictive residential setting with her financial affairs managed for her. The chair, on the hand, challenges the loss of independence and regressive direction planned for the future. Whilst acknowledging the risks, she upholds the ambitions of recovery and progress by advising the client to reconsider the direction being suggested. The client appears to accept the invitation. In both meetings, progress is being compromised by risks to the client, but the responsibilities are differently allocated. Both case meetings are concerned with progress and recovery, but with different responses.

So, principles of recovery and independence are undermined by risks. The workers might subscribe to these principles, but current risks take precedence. As Floersch (2002) notes, there is a difference between situated and disciplinary knowledge. Professional practices are directed by policies and procedures based on disciplinary ways of thinking, but these principles are enacted in situations where local knowledge and interpretations also have an influence: "Practitioners produce local, specific, contextual or situated knowledge in practice. Moreover, in contradistinction to the a priori disciplinary knowledge, these various conceptualisations see situated knowledge as dependent on activities or as knowledge in action." (Floersch 2002: 5–6).

Floersch (2002: 210) found that approaches promoted by policymakers and legislators had to be adapted by mental health case managers, but did not consider that this denoted resistance: "I do not think case managers' situated practice was subordinate to the state-mandated disciplinary power of strengths management." Similarly, Brodwin (2013: 49) found that another approach to case management, Assertive Community Treatment, involved case managers drawing on "infinite improvisation demanded by ordinary work". Workers and clients remain committed to ambitions such as progress and recovery, but risks get in the way.

Note

1 The example has been previously analysed from the point of view of clashing time discourses between the workers and the client in Juhila, Günther and Raitakari (2015) "Negotiating mental health rehabilitation plans: Joint future talk and clashing time talk in professional client Interaction", *Time & Society*, 24(1): 5–26.

References

Brodwin, P.E. (2013) *Everyday Ethics: Voices from the frontline of community psychiatry*, Berkeley: University of California Press.

Bull, R. and Shaw, I. (1992) "Constructing causal accounts in social work", *Sociology*, 26(4): 635–649.

Burns, T., Floritti, A., Holloway, F., Malm, U. and Rössler, W. (2001) "Case management and assertive community treatment in Europe", *Psychiatric Services*, 52(5): 631–636.

Clarke, J. (2006) "Consumerism and the remaking of state-citizen relations in the UK", in G. Marston and C. McDonald (eds) *Analysing Social Policy: A governmental approach* (pp. 89–106), Cheltenham, UK: Edward Elgar.

Coleman, R. (1999) *Recovery: An alien concept*, Gloucester, UK: Hansell Publishing.

Dall, T. and Caswell, D. (2015) "Interprofessional negotiation in multi-party interactions in social work", paper presented at the *DANASWAC conference*, Gent, 19 August 2015.

Dean, M. (1995) "Governing the unemployed self in an active society", *Economy and Society*, 24(4): 559–583.

Dean, M. (1999) "Risk, calculable and incalculable", in D. Lupton (ed.) *Risk and Sociocultural Theory: New directions and perspectives* (pp. 131–159), Cambridge: Cambridge University Press.

Department of Health (1990) *Caring for People: The care programme approach for people with a mental illness referred to specialist mental health services*, London: Department of Health.

Department of Health (2008) *Refocusing the Care Programme Approach*, London: Department of Health.

Ferguson, H. (2001) "Social work, individualization and life politics", *British Journal of Social Work*, 31(1): 41–55.

Ferguson, H. (2003) "In defence (and celebration) of individualization and life politics for social work", *British Journal of Social Work*, 33(5): 699–707.

Floersch, J. (2002) *Meds, Money and Manners: The case management of severe mental illness*, New York: Columbia University Press.

Foucault, M. (1991) "Governmentality", in G. Burchell, C. Gordon and P. Miller (eds) *The Foucault Effect: Studies in governmental rationality* (pp. 87–104), London: Harvester Wheatsheaf.

Freese, J. and Maynard, D. (1998) "Prosodic features of bad news and good news in conversation", *Language and Society*, 27(2): 195–219.

Garrett, P. (2003) "The trouble with Harry: why the new agenda of life politics fails to convince", *British Journal of Social Work*, 33(3): 381–397.

Garrett, P. (2004) "More trouble with Harry: a rejoinder in the 'life politics' debate", *British Journal of Social Work*, 34(4): 577–589.

Giddens, A. (1991) *Modernity and Self-Identity: Self and society in the late modern age*, Cambridge: Polity Press.

Giddens, A. (1999) "Risk and responsibility", *The Modern Law Review*, 62(1): 1–10.

Gould, D. (2013) *Service Users' Experiences of Recovery under the 2008 Care Programme Approach*, London: National Survivor User Network and the Mental Health Foundation.

Hall, C. and Slembrouck, S. (2001) "Parent participation in social work meetings: the case of child protection conferences", *European Journal of Social Work*, 4(2): 143–160.

Hitzler, S. and Messmer, H. (2010) "Group decision-making in child welfare and the pursuit of participation", *Qualitative Social Work*, 9(2): 205–226.

Holt, E. (1996) "Reporting on talk: the use of direct reported speech in conversation", *Research on Language and Social Interaction*, 29(3): 219–245.

Houston, S. (2004) "Garrett contra Ferguson: a meta theoretical appraisal of the 'rumble in the jungle'", *British Journal of Social Work*, 34(2): 261–267.

Juhila, K., Günther, K. and Raitakari, S. (2015) "Negotiating mental health rehabilitation plans: joint future talk and clashing time talk in professional client interaction", *Time & Society*, 24(1): 5–26.

Juhila, K., Jokinen, A. and Saario, S. (2014) "Reported speech", in C. Hall, K. Juhila, M. Matarese and C. van Nijnatten (eds) *Analysing Social Work Communication: Discourse in practice* (pp. 154–172), London: Routledge.

Kemshall, H. (2001) *Risk, Social Policy and Welfare*, Buckingham, UK: Open University Press.

Labov, W. (1972) *Language in the Inner City: Studies in the black English vernacular*, Pittsburgh: University of Pennsylvania Press.

Lupton, D. (1999) *Risk*, London: Routledge.

McKee, K. (2009) "Post-Foucauldian governmentality: what does it offer critical social policy analysis?", *Critical Social Policy*, 29(3): 465–486.

Nikander, P. (2003) "The absent client: case description and decision making in interprofessional meetings", in C. Hall, K. Juhila, N. Parton and T. Pösö (eds) *Constructing Clienthood in Social Work and Human Services: Interaction, identities and practices* (pp. 123–140), London: Jessica Kingsley Publishers.

Onyett, S. (1998) *Case Management in Mental Health*, London: Nelson Thornes.

Oxley, D. (2011) *Constructing Care in the Community Together: A discourse analysis of care planning meetings*, Unpublished doctoral thesis, University of East London.

Raitakari, S., Günther, K., Juhila, K. and Saario, S. (2013) "Causal accounts as a consequential device in categorizing mental health and substance abuse problems", *Communication & Medicine*, 10(3): 237–248.

Rose, N., O'Malley, P. and Valverde, M. (2006) "Governmentality", *Annual Review on
Law and Social Science*, 2: 83–104.

Sacks, H., Schegloff, E. and Jefferson, G. (1974) "A simplest systematics for the organization of turn-taking for conversation", *Language*, 50(4): 696–735.

Seing, I., Ståhl, C., Nordenfelt, L., Bülow, P. and Ekberg, K. (2012) "Policy and practice
of work ability: a negotiation of responsibility in organizing return to work", *Journal
of Occupational Rehabilitation*, 22(4): 553–564.

Simpson, A., Miller, C. and Bowers, L. (2003) "Case management models and the care
programme approach: how to make the CPA effective and credible", *Journal of Psychiatric and Mental Health Nursing*, 10(4): 472–483.

Welsh, M. (2014) "Resilience and responsibility: governing uncertainty in a complex
world", *The Geographical Journal*, 180(1): 15–26.

Wilińska, M. and Bülow, P. (2015) "The right feeling: emotions in the work rehabilitation process", paper presented at the *DANASWAC conference*, Gent, 19 August 2015.

Wooffitt, R. (1992) *Telling tales of Unexpected: The organization of factual discourse*,
Hemel Hempstead, UK: Harvester Wheatsheaf.

Part III

Managing worker and service provider responsibilities

8 Welfare workers reflecting their everyday responsibilities in focus groups

Jenni-Mari Räsänen and Sirpa Saario

Introduction

Responsibilities can be termed as the allocation of duties, obligations, jobs and tasks to individuals, groups and institutions (Martin 2007: 28–29; Fenwick 2016: 4). People can be, or be held, responsible for someone or something, and things can be done responsibly (Martin 2007: 28–29). Traditionally, responsibilities in workplaces are defined in contracts of employment but also in legislation and professional ethics (Iqbal *et al.* 2014: 27). When it comes to responsibilities of welfare workers, there are different interrelated and sometimes conflicting elements. Workers are noted to have to balance several obligations towards their clients, their employing organisation, their profession and broader society (Fenwick 2016: 8). Workers at the margins of welfare, such as mental health workers, are said to have little autonomy or control over their jobs, but they nevertheless "have responsibility for the most disabled and marginalised individuals" (Brodwin 2013: 3). They are also likely to face challenges between the desirable and the possible – testing whether their knowledge and training is enough to carry out appropriate decisions in demanding situations (Brodwin 2013: 29; see also Le Bianic 2011: 806).

In this chapter, we focus our attention on welfare workers' responsibilities from their own point of view. To put it more precisely, we examine how they reflect and make sense of their everyday responsibilities in focus groups. As Martin (2007: 23) notes, there are also mundane uses and definitions of responsibilities employed in the everyday settings. The workers whose reflections we focus on are employed by different mental health service providers. They have various occupational backgrounds, such as psychiatric nurses, practical nurses, occupational therapists and substance abuse workers. Nevertheless, they all perform rather similar work with their clients in the field of mental health and substance abuse. They work closely with their clients in their homes and/or supported housing services, and are in frequent face-to-face contact with their clients, unlike more specialised professionals. They provide support in everyday tasks of managing finances, household chores, independent living skills and social contacts.

Before examining focus group discussions, we discuss the welfare workers' responsibilities in relation to the managerialisation of welfare services and professional ethics. Following this, we approach these responsibilities through the concept of ethics work (Banks 2013) in order to emphasise the everyday aspects of responsibilities and how welfare workers balance between the macro-level demands and micro-level realities (Lipsky 1980; Maynard-Moody and Musheno 2003). By analysing workers' focus groups, we particularly illustrate how workers jointly account for the responsibilities relating to their various roles and duties in their everyday work with service users. Although responsibility and accountability are often seen from the policy-level perspective, there is also a need to approach them from the micro-level viewpoint – that is, how they are constructed and understood in the everyday talk and interactions of professionals (Matarese and Caswell 2014: 45–47).

Responsibilities and managerialisation of welfare services

The managerialisation of welfare services is recognised as a key challenge for welfare workers, as it affects their duties and responsibilities (Annandale 1996; Banks 2004; Henriksson *et al.* 2006; Juhila 2009: 300; Le Bianic 2011: 804; Chapter 2 of this volume). The managerialisation has meant the introduction of ideas from the private sector, meaning competition and contracts for services that focus on measurable outputs and outcomes, efficiency and effectiveness (Rajavaara 1993; Clarke and Newman 1997; Harris 2003; Juhila 2006; Connell *et al.* 2009; Banks 2013: 588). These changes have identified workers as "being personally held accountable for their own decisions and actions" (Le Bianic 2011: 804). For example, social workers are made responsible for "running the business" (Harris 2003: 66), but also they are "to be managed in the pursuit of government's policy agendas"; this has led workers to consider whether they are "doing the right things" or giving enough effort (Harris 2003: 182–183). Workers have faced demands to keep within budgets and to carry out productive, cost-effective, preventive or rehabilitative work (see Chapter 2). Related to this, workers are also increasingly required to produce quantifiable outcomes, and to be able to demonstrate they have followed and documented their performances, their tasks and certain procedures (Martin and Kettner 1997; Banks 2004: 152–153; Juhila 2006, 2009; Saario and Stepney 2009; Le Bianic 2011). This is called the *new accountability* (Banks 2004, 2013; Martin and Kettner 1997). Per-formances and outputs are more and more indicated via documents and informa-tion technology-based systems (Postle 2002; Parton 2008; Burton and van den Broek 2009; Juhila 2009: 301; Räsänen 2012; Saario 2014). It has been argued that, in particular, the welfare services contracted out to third-sector or private organisations face the demands of "performance measures" (Banks 2011: 11).

The changes in welfare services have meant "managerialist responsibilization of grass-roots level workers" (see Chapter 2). Responsibilisation is strongly associated with managerialism because it aims to render subjects responsible for tasks that previously would have been the duty of a state agency, or would have not even been recognised as a responsibility (O'Malley 2009: 277–279). The responsibilisation of workers can be seen to take place in two ways. First, traditionally workers can be seen as the subjects of responsibilisation where it is their responsibility to make their clients more responsible (e.g. Liebenberg *et al.* 2015) and to re-educate them (see Chapter 2). Second, workers can be seen as objects of responsibilisation where they themselves are made increasingly responsible for the contents and outcomes of services they deliver, as well as for assessing clients and delivering documents for administrative purposes (e.g. Le Bianic 2011). In other words, in the process of responsibilisation, welfare workers are both subjects and objects of responsibilisation, while state and local authorities become less involved in everyday work (see Chapter 2). Thus, grass-roots level workers are faced with balancing the demands of efficiency and the needs of their clients (Liebenberg *et al.* 2015: 1008).

It has been argued that the possibilities for professional discretion, e.g. having a command of the use of time and contacts with clients and the contents of work, have been reduced due to new managerialism requirements (Harris 2003: 74–75). Le Bianic (2011: 822) argues that as workers face the demands of certifying, verifying and validating certain facts or events, their expertise is characterised as being more "official" than discretionary. According to Brodkin (2008), this is problematic, particularly in social welfare work, where discretion is an essential part of the client–worker relationship. She notes how performance management may have unintended consequences for organisational performances, as although it may give the appearance of transparency and the illusion of accountability, in reality it obscures the full understanding of how the work is actually done in agencies, and what the real content and quality of the work is (Brodkin 2008: 323, 332). Hence, Brodkin (2008: 331–332) calls for research that examines how policies are produced and experienced in everyday practices (see also Hjörne *et al.* 2010). This resonates with the ethnomethodological idea of learning "seen, but unnoticed" features of talk and action (Garfinkel 1967: 41, 180).

Responsibilities and professional ethics

Responsibility relates to acting "in an ethical and accountable manner" (Giddens 1999: 8). Ethics is basically about how people "treat each other and their environment" and about the wrong and right character of action in different situations (Banks and Williams 2005: 1005). Professional ethics particularly relates to how professionals should act in certain situations, such as in relation to service users and what is expected of them (Banks and Williams 2005: 1005). Workers are expected to explain and justify their roles and duties as "who they are and what they have done or not done" (Banks 2013: 593), particularly in situations when there is a threat of being blamed for one's actions (Juhila 2009: 297). The ethical values of welfare workers are based on human rights and dignity as they are set responsibilities to act with integrity, compassion, empathy and care towards clients and patients (IFSW 2012; International Council of Nurses 2012; Talentia 2012). Banks and Gallagher (2009: 27) note how health and social care professionals share some main commonalities as to what counts as a good professional within these fields, such as being aware of their power and the vulnerability of those who are dependent on them. Also, the purpose of these professions is the promotion of welfare or social welfare at the individual and communal levels (Banks and Gallagher 2009: 18, 27). Professionals are also expected to know the ethical principles of their profession (Juhila and Raitakari 2010: 57; Fenwick 2016: 5–6), but are found to differ regarding their level of commitment to them (Metteri and Hotari 2011: 69).

Professional ethics can be regarded as not only rules and principles of conduct and action, but also as virtue-based approaches which shift attention towards professionals as "moral agents" who perceive salient features of each situation (Banks and Gallagher 2009: 213). Ethics thus involves constant reflection and dialogue (Metteri and Hotari 2011: 88). It has been argued that as normative guidelines, ethical codes cannot reach the details of work or remove the uncertainties workers face in practice (Brodwin 2013: 187). Dominelli and Holloway (2008: 1017) note how ethics as regulatory codes can "hold professionals to account for their behaviour", which also raises questions of to whom workers are actually accountable and how accountabilities are prioritised. Thus, workers need to use professional discretion, as ethical principles do not guarantee straightforward answers to everyday dilemmas (Juhila 2009: 309; Lipsky 1980; Evans 2011). Ethical discretion is said to be an essential part of professional practices that are framed with political, economic and moral demands (Talentia 2012: 11).

The promotion of empowerment and participation is essentially linked with the ethical being and acting in social welfare work (IFSW 2012; Talentia 2012), and are seen as important principles in community-based mental health services (Juhila and Raitakari 2010: 68; Chapter 3 of this volume). Empowerment-based work means taking clients or group of clients seriously "as experts of their own lives" (Simon 1994: 2). As a result, individuals are gradually able to improve their own lives and living conditions and are able to help themselves (see Chapter 3) and make their own choices and decisions (Videmšek 2014: 63). The emphasis on participation as a part of welfare policies has meant the need to increase the participation of citizens and service users in decision making and service delivery (Newman 2000: 55; Banks 2004: 41; Matthies 2014), as well as in planning their own services and individual recovery (see Chapter 6). As noted in Chapter 3, participation is regarded as an important right of citizens, and thus it is linked with professional expectations: "welfare workers are seen as responsible for encouraging, enabling and supporting them [clients] to use this right", for consulting and guiding clients in making choices about their services, and for informing them about the available options, as well as supporting them in their recovery processes. However, in reality, the ideas of participation may be threatened for many reasons, such as clients' complex needs or the ways services are delivered and provided (see Chapter 3). In the context of welfare services, participation should not be taken for granted, but there is a need for sensitive and bottom-up involvement of people (Matthies 2014: 15).

In this chapter, we regard the ethics of everyday work as a "matter of second thoughts" – reflections of workers' recent actions, such as what they just did or witnessed, what disturbed them or what their clients need (Brodwin 2013: 29). We analyse whether the organisational and political contexts "create boundaries for ethical being and acting" (Banks and Gallagher 2009: 214–216) among the welfare workers in question. As Mänttäri-van der Kuip (2013: 16, 2015) found out, the new accountability requirements of monitoring, evaluating and controlling of work may get workers into ethically contradictory situations, and has created a need for workers to balance contradictory interests in their everyday practices. Reamer (2006: 5, 44) notes that when professional values, duties, obligations and expectations of managerialism conflict, ethical dilemmas arise. Banks (2011: 19) suggests that ethical being and acting is a process that requires constant negotiation on what rules to notice, and to question what we are doing and why, but also requires "being alert to the dominance of the managerialist and neo-liberal agendas". Next we move on to analyse in more detail the ways welfare workers reflect upon and account for their everyday responsibilities.

Ethics work, responsibilities and accountability in focus groups

Analysing focus group talk

In order to analyse welfare workers' responsibilities, we utilise focus groups conducted with teams of workers. The workers in the interviews represent professions from a wide range of occupations in welfare services: psychiatric nurses, practical nurses, occupational therapists and substance abuse workers. Furthermore, there are also social care workers with varying vocational backgrounds ranging from task-based internal training courses to bachelor's degree qualifications in social care. Despite these diverse vocational backgrounds, focus groups aim to examine workers' shared reflections regarding their responsibilities, and thus create a more "general" picture of workers' accountability and the ways they perform the ethics work at the margins of welfare services.

The workers interviewed in six focus groups represent both supported housing and floating support services in Finland and England. The services are run by non-governmental organisations, which provide services for local authorities through a contractual tendering process (see Chapter 4). In line with current policies of deinstitutionalisation of welfare services, the settings provide care in the community, with the aim of facilitating the clients' meaningful life within their local communities. The supported housing services offer specialised housing, social rehabilitation and a home visiting service. These services differ regarding their target groups: some are aimed at a specialised group of clients with severe and co-occurring mental health and substance abuse problems, who are often termed as people with "dual diagnosis", whereas some have a more generic orientation and are intended for a wide range of people with mental health problems. The floating support services are intended for people with mental health problems, and offer mainly home visits to clients' own homes or client–worker meetings outside the home. The key working areas in both supported housing and floating support services focus on clients' everyday skills, social skills and medication as well as coping with illness or substance abuse.

Focus group interviews were designed to elicit workers' common talk where they can address various expectations and challenges they face as a team (see Morgan 2002). Analysis concentrates on the ways workers manage, account for or modify responsibilities in their everyday practices. We study responsibility from the micro-level viewpoint, and assess and draw conclusions as to whether or not the workers' talk on responsibilities actually reflects upon the managerialisation of welfare services and/or professional ethics (see Chapter 4). The frame for our analysis comes from Banks' (2016, 2013) notion of ethics work, which is per se a way of conceptualising the reasoning of the worker, and thus refers to cognitive elements of an individual person. Banks (2013) suggests that ethics work refers to situations where workers negotiate and balance tensions between their personal engagement and professional accountability. By personal engagement, Banks (2013: 590–593) refers basically to workers' motivations, value commitments and relationships with their clients, and to the processes of their everyday work and how they perform it. We utilise one particular dimension of ethics work: its interactional nature (see also Fenwick 2016: 7). We draw particularly on Banks' notion of ethics work as performance, where one puts on a performance of himself or herself as "doing ethics work" directed at other parties. As a performance, ethics work includes conversational moves that workers make during talk about "ethical aspects of situations, working out the right course of action and justifying who they are and what they have done" (Banks 2013: 599–600; see also Banks 2016: 45).

When analysing the empirical extracts from focus groups and the ethics work being performed in them, we apply the concepts of responsibility and accountability (see Chapter 4). These are closely connected in institutional encounters (Mäkitalo 2003: 496; Matarese and Caswell 2014: 47), and thus accounting for one's actions in these encounters also displays how responsibilities are carried out and talked into being (Matarese and Caswell 2014: 47). Responsibility is close to the idea of following the rules as achieved in action; they are not blindly followed, but are "realised and interpreted within and in relation to action" (Martin 2007: 23). Interviews are occasions full of accounts, and respondents are seen to account for their actions as competent members of a certain category (Baker 2003: 399). When workers are accounting for their actions, they are at the same time making visible their institutional tasks and problems related to them (Juhila *et al.* 2010: 75). Thus, the interviews provide opportunities for studying the ways workers are reflecting on their responsibilities.

According to Scott and Lyman (1968: 46), accounts "bridge the gap between actions and expectations". Accounting refers to the ways people explain, excuse and justify (Scott and Lyman 1968) their responsibilities or even blame themselves, other people or instances about troublesome issues or behaviour (Hall *et al.* 2006: 34; Chapter 4 of this volume). Scott and Lyman (1968: 46) conclude that when someone is *excusing* their behaviour they are mitigating or relieving their responsibility for the conduct in question. When they are *justifying* their behaviour, they are neutralising their conduct or act and its consequences, as the circumstances permit or require them to do so (Scott and Lyman 1968: 51). In ethnomethodology, accounting for one's action is seen more broadly as an inherent part of talk and interaction (Garfinkel 1967), as the participants of interaction constantly explain and make sense of their action (see Suoninen 1997; Baker 2003; Juhila *et al.* 2010).

The analysis concentrates on those instances in focus groups where workers talk about their responsibilities, and particularly on how they balance expectations arising from workers themselves and their clients, or those arising from managerial expectations. The empirical examples presented are closely connected to everyday work with clients, and illustrate how workers are accounting for their responsibilities in these situations. They differ from talk where workers reflect their responsibilities in relation to other practitioners and professional groups (see Chapter 9). We present five extracts that illustrate the following:

1   the ways workers are committing clients to take responsibility for themselves;
2   how workers regulate the amount of time and resources they provide to clients;
3   how workers balance between clients' privacy and getting their institutional tasks done during home visits;
4   how workers assess the amount and duration of home visits;
5   how workers try to comply with the performance measures.

Committing clients to take responsibility for themselves

The first extract is from a focus group with four workers from a Finnish supported housing service for people with mental health and substance abuse problems. Workers are talking about their responsibility for encouraging clients to be more committed to take responsibility for themselves.

Extract 1

1   INTERVIEWER: So, I'm asking what are the ways that you make [the clients] committed? [short laugh]
2   WORKER 4: Well, these discussions, I dunno whether they've had them before in [Supported housing service], at least nowadays, we have now.
3   WORKER 1: We have.
4   WORKER 2: Yeah, yeah. We have.
5   WORKER 1: Yeah, we have.
6   WORKER 4: So, will this continue, are you benefiting from this, or.... You don't have to be [here]. So, I have [said], well, this is not like in prison where you have to [unclear word] [short laugh], as if you don't get anything for yourself, 'cause you should be the one who benefits. Well, these kinds of ...

7   WORKER 1: We've had a lot of that [kind of discussions]. I've …
8   WORKER 4: Some are a bit amazed.
9   WORKER 3: Yeah, it's like, what are you talking about?
10   WORKER 2: Yeah, yeah.
11   WORKER 4: Something like that.
12   WORKER 2: Yeah, and you know it's not like, it is a kind of two-fold thing, 'cause there is no sense in putting people out of there, here, [everywhere] and then all over again. Still, to some extent you always have to do that.
13   WORKER 1: You have to.
14   WORKER 2: That either you commit yourself here and now, think about that for a while, when we give you some time to think about this, think how committed you are and then, but we won't then again throw [somebody] out of here when he's not committed again, but we have the same conversation again, and, well, that's how it is.
15   WORKER 1: Right, yes.
16   WORKER 3: Loosening and tightening.
17   WORKER 1: Yeah.

Just before the extract, worker 2 has been describing how it is the clients' responsibility to be committed but, on the other hand, how it is also the workers' responsibility to support the clients' commitment and to constantly reflect and monitor their engagement with the service. She justifies the importance of this kind of checking work, as it is easy for the client to say what s/he wants to achieve, but more difficult to know the ways and methods of achieving the goal. Her talk demonstrates that although clients are seen as responsible for their own conduct, the responsibility of professionals to support them is stronger.

The actual extract demonstrates collective and joint talk about client commitment and the ways the workers are reflecting it, as the interviewer poses a question: "*So, I'm asking what are the ways that you make [the clients] committed?*" (turn 1). The workers have contradictory thoughts about the issue, as the situations are case-specific and two-sided. Their responsibility is to get clients committed to their own responsibilities and objectives in rehabilitation. However, despite their efforts, the degree of commitment varies between clients (see also Ranta *et al.* 2016). The workers constantly have to reflect on this with their colleagues. Hence, they balance their own and clients' responsibilities. When negotiating the level of commitment with their clients, they compare and contrast their services to "*prison*" (turn 6) in order to display their clients' opportunities and freedom to make their own choices (see Chapter 3). In a way, they are relieving their responsibility (Scott and Lyman 1968: 47) and moving it partly to their clients (turn 6): "'*cause you should be the one who benefits*" and how some of the clients are "*amazed*" (turn 8) about this.

In turns 6 and 14–17, the workers are negotiating the process of commitment; they give time frames for clients to think about their level of commitment, but they do not "*throw them away*" if they are not committed. Thus, they do not abandon their clients, although there seems to be a constant balancing between loosening and tightening the client–worker relationship. They seem to be ensuring the stability of their clients (Brodwin 2013: 69) by trying to keep them in the supported housing services. The workers are doing the ethics work when they are negotiating the limits of helping – for example, considering whether they need to exceed or narrow their involvement when it comes to clients' commitment (Juhila and Raitakari 2010). The workers are assessing the right course of action and justifying their roles in this process (Banks 2013: 599–600). This also reflects the ethnomethodological view of responsibilities as being employed differently in everyday activities (Martin 2007: 33). Overall, this extract illustrates the ethical principle of responding to clients' needs (Juhila and Raitakari 2010: 68) and acting in an ethically responsible way as a work team.

Regulating the amount of time and resources

In the second extract, interviewers and three workers from an English supported housing and floating support service are talking about the use of working hours per client, and how workers negotiate and balance their use of time in practice. There are two interviewers and four workers present in the interview.

Extract 2

1 INTERVIEWER 1: How about, if they [clients] contact you, what do you do if you have used your four hours, let's say, and then somebody rings up, and you have a phone call, it's over your hour? [a short laugh] Do you say that, we don't have more time this week, let's talk about next week or, what do you …

2 WORKER 4: Depends on the situation.

3 WORKER 1: If it's serious, then you'll give …

4 WORKER 4: The [unclear word], in our case. In case [unclear word] quite serious, it would be heartless not to offer.

5 INTERVIEWER 1: Yeah, to respond in a sense.

6 WORKER 4: More support.

7 WORKER 1: If they're in a crisis situation, we do come out to them. And deal with it.

8 WORKER 3: I suppose, it's using your own discretion isn't it, whether it …

9 WORKER 1: [unclear word] client as well, what they like, and, if they're likely to ring, and ask for more support when they actually don't need it.

10 WORKER 3: Yeah. [a short laugh]

11 INTERVIEWER 2: And that's, I mean, I know you've got to keep very detailed records of your hours.

12 WORKER 1: Yeah.

13 INTERVIEWER 2: But within that you can, [unclear word] extra?

14 WORKER 1: Yeah.

15 WORKER 4: If you want to, yes. Wouldn't have to go too high in the manage-
        ment chain, to get that together. But we do it often.
16 WORKER 1: 'Cause I have taken someone to the doctor before, and, I've
        ended up being hours there. You couldn't leave because, it's kind of
        important there and then. I just told people that I was gonna be longer,
        that I would not go.
17 WORKER 2: And I've been on a visit and found out that, the lady I was with
        had taken an overdose, and I had to take her to hospital, and I was....
        So, I couldn't leave until the crisis team came, took over my role.
        'Cause she's on her own, in case she tried to get out and ...
18 INTERVIEWER 2: So in that case, what, I mean, are hours found from some-
        where or, is it just ...
19 WORKER 2: Yeah, it's generally. In that circumstance I contact my manager
        and say, this has happened, I'm gonna go to hospital with her. And
        they'll say that's fine, and then they just [unclear word] explained,
        what's happened and why that person's had the extra hours.

The extract starts with the interviewer's question about the use of time with each
client: what workers ought to do if a client calls and they have already received
their allotted hours. Earlier in the interview, it came out that the workers are able
to spend four hours with each client per week. Workers jointly describe these
situations as case-specific and the kind that needs their attention if they are
serious. Also, in turn 4, worker 4 notes if the situation is serious it would be
"*heartless not to offer*" support, which reflects strong personal engagement with
their work. At turn 7, worker 1 continues that if a client is in a crisis situation
they just "*deal with it*"; it is their responsibility. At turn 8, worker 3 produces an
indirect question of whether these are situations where they use their own discretion. Then at turn 9, worker 1 notes how their clients are also made responsible
for reflecting upon their situation: whether their situation is serious enough to
call for the service.

At turn 11, interviewer 2 asks about the detailed recording of working hours
the workers have "*got to keep*", and whether they can do something extra within
the given time frame. Worker 4 says that they do not need to ask permission
from high management in order to do that (turn 15). Then in turns 16 and 17,
workers 1 and 2 justify the use of extra time in certain situations by giving concrete examples. They describe situations when they have used discretion and
exceeded the four hours per client. Those have been situations where they
"*couldn't leave*", which emphasises their seriousness. Their talk reflects how
clients' well-being is their first priority.

Interviewer 2 is interested in whether the time is taken away from something
else (turn 18). Worker 2 responds that they just contact their manager, and give
an explanation of what has happened and why the extra hours have been used.
According to her, the manager is fine with this. Within the given time frames,
they are able to regulate their use of time if they have grounds for it. Thus, the
workers obviously have space and opportunity for case-specific discretion (see

Evans 2011). This extract illustrates how the workers are doing ethics work, as they case-specifically regulate the duration of time and resources with their clients and negotiate what rules to apply and why in each situation (see also Chapter 10). They are working out the right course of action from the client's point of view (Banks 2013: 599–600). This extract also shows the workers' responsibility for the most marginalised people (Brodwin 2013: 3).

Balancing between clients' privacy and institutional tasks during home visits

In the third extract, four workers from a Finnish floating support service for people with mental health problems are talking with the interviewer about the professional way of doing home visits, and how workers are constantly balancing clients' privacy and their institutional responsibilities:

Extract 3

1 INTERVIEWER: OK. Let's move on to home visiting, as a working arena. How does it appear to you?

2 WORKER 1: Maybe it's in a way more free, if you compare it to [nursing home], as, well, as an example, like the level of cleanliness I've said before somewhere that, in [nursing home] there are certain things you have to clean and, when, and which day, but in one's own home it's not – it doesn't have to be so tidy necessarily. Maybe the home is then also more unpredictable, as you never know what you're up against when you enter, like are there other people, what has happened, these kinds of things.

3 WORKER 3: And the point that it's done quite a lot on the client's terms then, as you certainly can't ...

4 WORKER 1: Yeah, sure.

5 WORKER 3: ... evaluate that level of cleanliness or other things as it's his/her home and just the way it is. Certainly, you can always talk and negotiate about it, but it's not our purpose to go there to evaluate it. It's precisely that encounter when you ring the doorbell, it's already the moment when the client comes to the door that you already evaluate it, the fluency of the visit and how it's perhaps going to be or ...

6 WORKER 1: Yes, it is.

7 WORKER 3: ... so, it's rather interesting.

8 WORKER 1: Or if the client wants you to leave right away, that you have to leave, so, we have to leave then, it's not our, it's not me who ... [laughing].

9 WORKER 4: Yes, you constantly have to remember that we're in the client's own home, and kind of evaluate that you won't cross the line of self-determination then.

10 WORKER 2: Yes, I think it's very respectful.

11 WORKER 4: Yes.

12   WORKER 2: The starting point is that the client decides when the visit kind of ends, or do we stick to what's been agreed, or does he/she let us in, so anyway it starts with that. But you still can't forget your professional competence, so, this co-operation is based on us coming with respect, but we're here for the reason that some form of co-operation is agreed on, rehabilitative relationship, that we're not just visiting either.

13   WORKER 1: Mm.

14   WORKER 4: Mm.

15   WORKER 3: Mm.

16   WORKER 2: So that kind of, and then there is the self-determination that you have to respect, but it remains the whole time.

17   WORKER 4: And then, well?

18   WORKER 3: So I think that the home tells a lot.

19   WORKER 1: Mm-m.

20   WORKER 3: There's so much information when you enter there and opens up in front of our eyes so that ...

21   WORKER 4: Yeah.

22   WORKER 1: Yes.

23   WORKER 3: You can see so much about the client's strengths, and how the home perhaps changes during the journey, you can make a lot of conclusions already based on that, and make observations.

24   WORKER 4: Yes, and then if you think, what's the worker's view on something, like on a clean home or a healthy diet, so anyway it's not the same – what is the client's view and what's exactly true for the client, the client's, so in a way you must, at some point, give up a little and accept that OK, this is the client's home and his/her view.

25   WORKER 3: Certainly I think that in an extreme case – well, we have to put it into words if the home appears ...

26   WORKER 2: Of course, absolutely.

In this extract, the interviewer starts with a question about home visiting and how it appears to the workers. Worker 1 starts to compare home visiting with working at a nursing home, which had stricter rules and timetables regarding the level of cleanliness in comparison with working at clients' own homes. She also notes how the home appears to her as a more unpredictable place than a nursing home. Then the discussion continues with worker 3's notion of conducting home visits on clients' own terms. The workers can negotiate and talk about cleaning with their clients, but their duty is not to evaluate the level of cleanliness. Cleaning seems to be quite a delicate issue. Worker 3 describes how the first contact with a client at his or her door says much about the forthcoming encounter. Worker 1 confirms this at turn 6: "*Yes it is*". The workers' dialogue reflects their professional know-how and intuition. At turn 8, worker 1 notes the importance of respecting clients' own will and power: if they want a worker to leave, then they have to leave and respect it. Worker 4 continues that they constantly need to remember that they are in a client's private space, their home, and they need to respect his or her self-determination.

At turn 12, worker 2 describes how home visits need to be very respectful, and how they need to take into account the client's needs and wishes. Nevertheless, she notes their professional responsibility: as they cannot forget their professional competence and the original idea behind the support relationship and home visiting. She distinguishes their visits from "normal" visiting, and justifies their responsibility to comply with the agreement and the clients' rehabilitation. Other workers support her account. Then, again, worker 2 returns to comments on the respect for clients' self-determination, which is always present when they are visiting clients' homes (turn 16). Worker 3 continues to justify the importance of home visits in their work, as they tell them a lot about the client's situation and produce important information for them. Then worker 4 comes back to the issue of cleaning, how workers' and clients' perceptions about a clean house or healthy diet may differ, and how workers need to distinguish their own way of thinking from the client's way of perceiving these issues (turn 24). Worker 3 justifies their responsibility to nevertheless "*put it into words*" if there is some serious trouble or deficiency in the client managing at home. Their institutional tasks in some circumstances permit or require them to do so (Scott and Lyman 1968: 51).

This extract displays the workers' subtle practices as they are constantly striking a balance between respecting clients' privacy and self-determination and conducting their institutional tasks of checking up on the client and his or her everyday coping during the home visits. The workers' responsibility is to work out the right course of action, and they need to justify their roles in regard to who they are and what they will do (see Banks 2013: 599–600) during the home visits. They need to be sensitive when making their judgements e.g. about cleaning, but their duty is also to comment if they notice that the home does not correspond sufficiently to "normal" living standards (see also Räsänen and Saario 2015).

Assessing the amount and duration of home visits

Our fourth example is from the same interview as Extract 1. Here the workers and the interviewer are talking about the amount and duration of home visits.

Extract 4

1   WORKER 4: Yes, and also at the moment we think, for real, that when we make home visits [in supported housing service], they can't all last for an hour or 45 minutes, it sometimes may be only half an hour or even 15 minutes for someone. Well, it shows from the client then, how much he/she can handle it.

2   WORKER 2: For [a certain client] it's sometimes eight minutes when he started to say …

3   WORKER 4: Yeah, right, that one.

4   WORKER 2: … that I believe this was it, well, then we try to hang out for another eight minutes, as we don't usually leave there much before a quarter of an hour, but …

5   INTERVIEWER: Do you have permission to visit everyone's home?
6   WORKER 2: Yes, we require it.
7   WORKER 1: Yeah, yes, it's, we visit everyone, but then again we don't visit everyone at the moment. But it's the municipality's wish, that we make visits for everyone, and they are interested in how often we visit there.
8   WORKER 3: And we make it individually once a week for someone, twice a week for another, or then once a month.

The extract starts with worker 4's description of the practices of home visits in the supported housing services. She mentions the time limit of 45 minutes to one hour, which evidently refers to the expected length of home visits instructed by the municipality. She then explains how, in practice, the visits do not necessarily last that long. She justifies this with the client's condition and how long a visit they can handle. She portrays herself and her colleagues as experts in estimating the client's individual condition and needs, and how longer visits may even have a negative effect on the client's situation. They possess "everyday evidence" (Saario *et al.* 2015; Chapter 9 of this volume) of a client's situation that the purchaser is lacking. Worker 2 gives the example of a client for whom eight minutes was long enough, and describes how she and her colleague nevertheless stay at his home for another eight minutes, because they try to stay at least 15 minutes at each visit. Thus, they act in accordance with a certain time limit.

In turn 5, the interviewer asks whether the workers have permission to visit every home. Worker 2 answers that they require it. In turn 7, worker 1 continues that the responsibility to visit every client's home comes from the municipality that purchases the service. Nevertheless, worker 1's talk in this turn indicates that the workers are not obliged to do so, as it is the municipality's "*wish*" that the workers visit every home, and they are "*interested in*" the amount of visits they make. She says that "*we visit everyone, but then again we don't visit everyone at the moment*". Her talk hints that they are modifying the municipality's expectations to fit with their everyday work. They also have space and opportunities for case-sensitive discretion: "*we make it individually once a week for someone, twice a week for another, or then once a month*". The workers' dialogue demonstrates how the responsibility to visit clients regularly at home and for a certain amount of time does not necessarily work in practice; they are thus mediating between macro-level resources and micro-level realities (Lipsky 1980). The workers are sensitive to clients' needs and capabilities to participate and to make their own choices regarding their services (see Chapter 3; Videmšek 2014: 63). Overall, the ethics work is manifested when the workers do not literally comply with the managerial expectations, but instead they balance different interests and act in a case-sensitive way (see Banks 2011, 2013; Mänttäri-van der Kuip 2013, 2015; Liebenberg *et al.* 2015).

Trying to comply with performance measures

Our last extract is from another focus group with welfare workers from a Finnish supported housing service. Before the extract, the workers have been discussing the nature and form of personal contacts and what should be counted as a personal contact. In the following extract, three workers are talking about changes in recording practices and in the monitoring of their work performance. Five welfare workers and two interviewers are present in the interview.

Extract 5

1   WORKER 1: And then, here's this kind of, at least what I've been thinking about. As now there's this message coming from [commissioning agency] that they follow, that those need to be seen there, these personal contacts or home visits, they need to be seen there on the computer. So, in a way it has probably increased our efforts to try so hard now, a bit too slavishly to comply, so it's like, whether it is the personal contact here [at the supported housing unit] or [unclear talk], so you constantly think of what you roughly record, so, OK [the person from the commissioning agency] is going to read these tomorrow [laughing].
2   WORKER 2: Yes, they give [that impression].
3   WORKER 1: But they have communicated to us that they'll follow them all the time and that they are realised as well.
4   WORKER 3: And this is just recording all the time.
5   WORKER 1: Yes, it has increased a lot.
6   WORKER 3: Before this tendering, we recorded once a week [some unclear talk], haa [is tapping on the desk] I have that many personal visits at the moment [laughing].

This extract starts with worker 1's description of the "*message*" that has come from the commissioning agency regarding the need to record personal contacts and/or home visits. She wonders whether they comply with these new instructions too "*slavishly*" in their everyday work. Nevertheless, these new responsibilities have caused a concern about whether they are recording enough, and recording the right issues (turn 1): "*whether it is the personal contact here [at the supported housing unit] or [unclear talk] so you constantly think of what you roughly record*". The pressure for recording comes from the potential audience of their records (Askeland and Payne 1999), which in this case is from the commissioning agency. In turn 3, worker 1 continues that they were given an impression that their recordings will be monitored. Then from turn 5 the workers bring out the growing amount of recording work and how it has increased since the tendering process. They used to record only once per week, but this has changed remarkably.

This extract demonstrates how the managerialisation of welfare services has an influence on welfare workers' responsibilities. The workers have faced the new accountability requirements of performance measures as the amount of recording work has increased; they have a responsibility to demonstrate the outputs (personal contacts) of work, and they need to be able to follow and document these outputs in certain ways (e.g. Banks 2004: 152–153). The workers' dialogue reflects the ethics work in the sense that they are working out what to record, and why and how this new situation has caused concerns and pressures for them as the amount and content of their work will be, at least potentially, monitored.

Conclusion and discussion

In this chapter we have analysed five extracts that illustrate the ways the workers are reflecting on their responsibilities in mental health supported housing and floating support services in Finland and England. The empirical examples are closely related to everyday work with clients. Workers are reflecting on their responsibility to encourage clients to be committed to their own responsibilities. They also discuss their need to negotiate between clients' privacy and getting their institutional task of checking and following the clients' well-being and everyday coping done during the home visits. Welfare workers also reflect on their responsibility to regulate the amount of time and resources they can offer for their clients. They also discuss how they try to comply with changes in recording practices and the monitoring of their work performance. Such practices indicate that workers are constantly doing "ethics work" as they take responsibility for being ethical and acting ethically (Banks 2016: 45–46). The practices resemble Brodwin's (2013: 29) findings on mental health workers' everyday ethics; these are reflections of actions and things that have disturbed workers, and which are related to their clients' needs. It is crucial that these welfare workers have "responsibility for the most disabled and marginalized individuals" and the responsibility to ensure their stability (Brodwin 2013: 3, 69), which is challenged by the changing conditions of their work.

Our aim was to examine and demonstrate how welfare workers talk into being the expectations coming from both the managerialisation of welfare services and professional ethics. It is obvious that welfare workers are expected to balance efficiency with clients' case-specific needs (Liebenberg *et al.* 2015: 1008). Workers have new responsibilities, and they are in this sense objects of responsibilisation (e.g. Le Bianic 2011); for example, they are expected to make a certain number of home visits and to report the time they have spent with their clients. In addition, these new accountability requirements are evident when workers reflect on trying to comply with the growing amount of recording work and the possibility that their work performances will be monitored through these recordings. Even so, the workers' talk regarding their everyday responsibilities also reflects that they are subjects of responsibilisation (e.g. Liebenberg *et al.* 2015). Workers make their clients responsible for assessing their level of commitment, which resonates with the findings from mental health case files where clients are held accountable for their progress and recovery, and how help could only be given for those who are ready to receive it (Liebenberg *et al.* 2015: 1016).

The workers' interview talk reflects everyday ethics work in the sense that ethical issues are constantly discussed, even though the word "ethics" is not used (Juhila and Raitakari 2010: 68). The extracts demonstrate and make visible how workers are performing ethics work as they are balancing and working out the right course of actions and justifying their roles and duties (Banks 2013: 599–600). Although the workers in the interviews do not represent the strong professions, they nevertheless have space and opportunity to develop "frontline versions" of managerial expectations. According to Lipsky (1980), discretion is essential for street-level bureaucrats to make policies work (Evans 2011: 370). In their focus group talk, workers frequently describe how they use case-sensitive discretion, and how they give priority to clients' well-being and safety despite the time limits and resources they could "officially" offer. Thus, when workers are faced with conflicting expectations, they prioritise their clients' needs and well-being.

During home visits, the welfare workers' task is to check up on the client and their everyday coping, but at the same time they need to respect clients' own territory and wishes. This is similar to the findings from home visit interactions, where workers are managing their identities as a guest and as a professional (Juhila *et al.* 2016). Conducting home visits and entering clients' private spaces calls for ethical sensitiveness and continuous discretion from workers. When necessary, they negotiate the limits of helping – whether there is a need to narrow or exceed their help towards clients (see Juhila and Raitakari 2010: 69). They are promoting participation and empowerment when they are sensitive to clients' wishes and capabilities to make their own choices regarding their services and commitment. Overall, workers' talk reflects how they are aware of their power and of their clients' vulnerability (Banks and Gallagher 2009).

In welfare services, responsibilities relate closely to accountability (Fournier 1999; Le Bianic 2011: 804). Workers have traditionally been held accountable for their decisions and actions in relation to different stakeholders, such as colleagues, employers and clients, and in relation to legislation (Banks 2004; Hall *et al.* 2006: 16; Juhila 2009) and ethical codes (Juhila 2009: 297; IFSW 2012; Talentia 2012; International Council of Nurses 2012). The welfare workers' everyday responsibilities presented in the extracts show that their accountabilities indeed unfold in different directions (Juhila 2009: 298). In our view, the accounts given by the welfare workers in the focus groups are close to Juhila's (2009: 304–306) notion of critical accountability, which she recognises as an important counterforce for the new accountability requirements. According to her, it challenges workers to do the following:

- to recognise and articulate the impossibilities and boundaries of their work tasks;
- to recognise the difficulties in measuring and standardising their work;
- to accept that professional discretion and human judgement are part of their everyday work.

In the focus groups analysed in this chapter, welfare workers reflect all these elements. Critical accountability is demonstrated especially in three responsibilities that workers reflect and comment on: regulating the amount of time and resources, assessing the amount and duration of home visits, and complying with the increasing amount of recording work.

Although it is not apparent in the selected interview extracts, it has been observed that when workers have little opportunity to influence their work, it may prevent them from doing client-centred work and may cause them work-related stress and anxiety (Tainio and Wrede 2008: 190). When it comes to studying workers' responsibilities, it is also essential to consider the differences in status and opportunities between different occupational groups, and how some groups may be left vulnerable in relation to others (Henriksson *et al.* 2006: 183). When the duties and tasks assigned to different professional groups (some more specialised than others) differ, they are also likely to set certain boundaries between their competences and responsibilities (see Chapter 9).

References

Annandale, E. (1996) "Working on the front-line: risk culture and nursing in the new NHS", *The Sociological Review*, 44(3): 416–451.

Askeland, G.A. and Payne, M. (1999) "Authors and audiences: towards a sociology of case recording", *European Journal of Social Work*, 2(1): 55–65.

Baker, C. (2003) "Ethnomethodological analyses of interviews", in J.A. Holstein and J.F. Gubrium (eds) *Inside Interviewing: New lenses, new concerns* (pp. 395–412), London: Sage.

Banks, S. (2004) *Ethics, Accountability and the Social Professions*, Basingstoke, UK: Palgrave Macmillan.

Banks, S. (2011) "Ethics in an age of austerity: social work and evolving new public management", *Journal of Social Intervention: Theory and Practice*, 20(2): 5–23.

Banks, S. (2013) "Negotiating personal engagement and professional accountability: professional wisdom and ethics work", *European Journal of Social Work*, 16(5): 587–604.

Banks, S. (2016) "Everyday ethics in professional life: social work as ethics work", *Ethics and Social Welfare*, 10(1): 35–52.

Banks, S. and Gallagher, A. (2009) *Ethics in Professional Life: Virtues for health and social care*, Basingstoke, UK: Palgrave Macmillan.

Banks, S. and Williams, R. (2005) "Accounting for ethical difficulties in social welfare work: issues, problems and dilemmas", *British Journal of Social Work*, 35(7): 1005–1022.

Brodkin, E. (2008) "Accountability in street-level organizations", *International Journal of Public Administration*, 31(3): 317–336.

Brodwin, P.E. (2013) *Everyday Ethics: Voices from the frontline of community psychiatry*, Berkeley: University of California Press.

Burton, J. and van den Broek, D. (2009) "Accountable and countable: information management systems and the bureaucratization of social work", *British Journal of Social Work*, 39(7): 1326–1342.

Clarke, J. and Newman, J. (1997) *Managerial State: Power, politics and ideology in the remaking of social welfare*, London: Sage.

Connell, R., Fawcett, B. and Meagher, G. (2009) "Neoliberalism, NPM and the human service professions", *Journal of Sociology*, 45(4): 331–338.

Dominelli, L. and Holloway, M. (2008) "Ethics and governance in social work research in the UK", *British Journal of Social Work*, 38(5): 1009–1024.

Evans, T. (2011) "Professionals, managers and discretion: critiquing street-level bureaucracy", *British Journal of Social Work*, 41(2): 368–386.

Fenwick, T. (2016) *Professional Responsibility and Professionalism: A sociomaterial examination*, London: Routledge.

Fournier, V. (1999) "The appeal to professionalism as a disciplinary mechanism", *The Sociological Review*, 47(2): 280–307.

Garfinkel, H. (1967) *Studies in Ethnomethodology*, Cambridge: Polity Press.

Giddens, A. (1999) "Risk and responsibility", *The Modern Law Review*, 62(1): 1–10.

Hall, C., Slembrouck, S. and Sarangi, S. (2006) *Language Practices in Social Work: Categorisation and accountability in child welfare*, London: Routledge.

Harris, J. (2003) *The Social Work Business*, London: Routledge.

Henriksson, L., Wrede, S. and Burau, V. (2006) "Understanding professional projects in welfare service work: revival of old professionalism?", *Gender, Work and Organisation*, 13(2): 174–192.

Hjörne, E., Juhila, K. and van Nijnatten, C. (2010) "Negotiating dilemmas in the practices of street-level welfare work", *International Journal of Social Welfare*, 19(3): 303–309.

IFSW (2012) *Statement of Ethical Principles*, International Federation of Social Workers, retrieved 16 October 2015 from http://ifsw.org/policies/statement-of-ethical-principles/.

International Council of Nurses (2012) *The ICN Codes of Ethics for Nurses*, Geneva: International Council of Nurses.

Iqbal, N., Reese, M. and Backer, C. (2014) "Decision making, responsibility and accountability in community mental health teams", *Mental Health Practice*, 17(7): 26–28.

Juhila, K. (2006) *Sosiaalityöntekijöinä ja asiakkaina: Sosiaalityön yhteiskunnalliset tehtävät ja paikat* [As social workers and clients: The societal functions and places of social work], Tampere: Vastapaino.

Juhila, K. (2009) "Sosiaalityön selontekovelvollisuus" [Accountability in social work], *Janus*, 17(4): 296–312.

Juhila, K. and Raitakari, S. (2010) "Ethics in professional interaction: justifying the limits of helping in a supported housing unit", *Ethics and Social Welfare*, 4(1): 57–71.

Juhila, K., Hall, C. and Raitakari, S. (2010) "Accounting for the clients' troublesome behaviour in a supported housing unit: blames, excuses and responsibility in professionals' talk", *Journal of Social Work*, 10(1): 59–79.

Juhila, K., Hall, C. and Raitakari, S. (2016) "Interaction during mental health floating support home visits: managing host-guest and professional-client identities in home spaces", *Social & Cultural Geography*, 17(1): 101–119.

Le Bianic, T. (2011) "Certified expertise and professional responsibility in organisations: the case of mental health practice in prisons", *The Sociological Review*, 59(4): 803–827.

Liebenberg, L., Ungar, M. and Ikeda, J. (2015) "Neo-liberalism and responsibilisation in the discourse of social service workers", *British Journal of Social Work*, 45(3), 1006–1021.

Lipsky, M. (1980) *Street-level Bureaucracy: Dilemmas of the individual in public services*, New York: Russell Sage Foundation.

Martin, D. (2007) "Responsibility: a philosophical perspective", in G. Dewsbury and J. Dobson (eds) *Responsibility and Dependable Systems* (pp. 21–42), London: Springer.

Martin, L.L. and Kettner, P.M. (1997) "Performance measurement: the new accountability", *Administration in Social Work*, 21(1): 17–29.

Matarese, M. and Caswell, D. (2014) "Accountability", in C. Hall, K. Juhila, M. Matarese and C. Van Nijnatten (eds) *Analysing Social Work Communication: Discourse in practice* (pp. 44–60), London: Routledge.

Matthies, A.-L. (2014) "How participation, marginalization and welfare services are interconnected", in A.-L. Matthies and L. Uggerhøj (eds) *Participation, Marginalization and Welfare Services: Concepts, politics and practices across European countries* (pp. 3–18), Surrey: Ashgate.

Maynard-Moody, S. and Musheno, M. (2003) *Cops, Teachers, Counselors: Stories from the front lines of public service*, Ann Arbor: University of Michigan Press.

Metteri, A. and Hotari, K.-E. (2011) "Eettinen kuormittuminen ja toimintaympäristö nuorten palveluissa" [Ethical burdening and operational context in the services for young people], in A. Pehkonen and M. Väänänen-Fomin (eds) *Sosiaalityön arvot ja etiikka* [Values and ethics in social work] (pp. 67–92), Jyväskylä, Finland: PS-Kustannus.

Morgan, D. (2002) "Focus group interviewing", in J.F. Gubrium and J.A. Holstein (eds) *Handbook of Interview Research: Context & method* (pp. 141–159), Thousand Oaks, CA: Sage.

Mäkitalo, Å. (2003) "Accounting practices and situated knowing: dilemmas and dynamics in institutional categorization", *Discourse Studies*, 5(4): 495–516.

Mänttäri-van der Kuip, M. (2013) "Julkinen sosiaalityö markkinoistumisen armoilla?" [Public social work at the mercy of marketization?], *Yhteiskuntapolitiikka*, 78(1): 5–19.

Mänttäri-van der Kuip, M. (2015) *Work-Related Well-being among Finnish Frontline Social Workers in an Age of Austerity*, Jyväskylä, University of Jyväskylä.

Newman, J. (2000) "Beyond the new public management? Modernizing public services", in J. Clarke, S. Gewirtz and E. McLaughlin (eds) *New Managerialism, New Welfare?* (pp. 45–61), London: Sage.

O'Malley, P. (2009) "Responsibilization", in A. Wakefield and J. Fleming (eds) *The SAGE Dictionary of Policing* (pp. 277–279), London: Sage.

Parton, N. (2008) "Changes in the form of knowledge in social work: from the 'social' to the 'informational'?", *British Journal of Social Work*, 38(2): 253–269.

Postle, K. (2002) "Working 'between the idea and the reality': ambiguities and tensions in care managers' work", *British Journal of Social Work*, 32(3): 335–351.

Rajavaara, M. (1993) "Markkinaohjautuvuus sosiaalityön haasteena" [Market orientation as a challenge for social work], in S. Karvinen and P. Aho (eds) *Sosiaalityön eettiset jännitteet* [Ethical dilemmas in social work] (pp. 63–73), Helsinki: Sosiaalityöntekijäin liitto r.y.

Ranta, J., Raitakari, S. and Juhila, K. (2016) "Rajatyö ja vastuut huumeidenkäyttäjien asunnottomuuden toiminnallisissa loukuissa" [Boundary work and responsibilities in the double binds of drug users' homelessness], Unpublished manuscript.

Reamer, F.G. (2006) *Social Work Values and Ethics*, New York: Columbia University Press.

Räsänen, J.-M. (2012) "Accounting for IT-based use of information in emergency social work encounters", *Nordic Social Work Research*, 2(1): 21–37.

Räsänen, J.-M. and Saario, S. (2015) "Telecare as institutional interaction: checking up on the client and creating continuity", *Journal of Technology in Human Services*, 33(3): 205–224.

Saario, S. (2014) *Audit Techniques in Mental Health: Practitioners' responses to electronic health records and service purchasing agreements*, Tampere: Acta Universitatis Tamperensis, 1907.

Saario, S. and Stepney, P. (2009) "Managerial audit and community mental health: a study of rationalizing practices in Finnish psychiatric outpatient clinics", *European Journal of Social Work*, 12(1): 41–56.

Saario, S., Juhila, K. and Raitakari, S. (2015) "Boundary work in inter-agency and inter-professional client transitions", *Interprofessional Journal of Care*, 29(6): 610–615.

Scott, M. and Lyman, S. (1968) "Accounts", *American Sociological Review*, 33(1): 46–62.

Simon, B.L. (1994) *The Empowerment Tradition in American Social Work: A history*, New York: Columbia University Press.

Suoninen, E. (1997) "Selonteot ja oman toiminnan ymmärrettäväksi tekeminen" [Accounts and making sense of one's action], *Sosiologia, 34(1): 26–38.*

Tainio, L. and Wrede, S. (2008) "Practical nurses' work role and workplace ethos in an era of austerity", in S. Wrede, L. Henriksson, H. Høst, S. Johansson and B. Dybbroe (eds) *Care Work in Crisis: Reclaiming the Nordic ethos of care* (pp. 177–198), Lund: Studenlitteratur.

Talentia (2012) *Arki, arvot, elämä ja etiikka: sosiaalialan ammattilaisen eettiset ohjeet* [Everyday living, values, life and ethics: ethical guidelines for social welfare workers], Talentia, Union of Professional Social Workers, Helsinki: Committee on Professional Ethics, retrieved 15 May 2016 from www.talentia.fi/files/558/Etiikkaopas_2013_net. pdf.

Videmšek, P. (2014) "From definition to action: empowerment as a tool for change in social work practice", in A.-L. Matthies and L. Uggerhøj (eds) *Participation, Marginalization and Welfare Services: Concepts, politics and practices across European countries* (pp. 63–76), Surrey: Ashgate.

9 Negotiating boundaries of professional responsibilities in team meetings

Sirpa Saario, Jenni-Mari Räsänen and Christopher Hall

Introduction

Legislation and organisational procedures regarding social and health care define the responsibilities of health and welfare workers. For example, decisions on hospital admissions are carried out by the psychiatrist in charge of the client, placements for supported housing are ultimately approved by the municipal commissioner, and everyday face-to-face contact with the client is maintained by the support worker. Despite these official and apparently clear-cut duties, the operation of mundane care work often gives workers uncertainty regarding their roles and expectations (Thompson and Dowding 2001; Tainio and Wrede 2008). For example, Iqbal *et al.* (2014) report many unresolved debates on how mental health workers should proceed with their clients. Therefore, often responsibilities are ultimately shaped in everyday negotiations that Håland (2012: 768) characterises as "interactions that are not fixed and predetermined but that are dependent upon interpretations, discussions and contexts". Slembrouck and Hall (2014: 64) note that negotiations on boundaries of responsibilities take place in professional interaction where participants are sorting out "who will do what" and "who is, or should be, responsible for what". Scourfield (2015) calls this "negotiated reality", which refers to the ambiguity regarding who is responsible for making, implementing and checking up on various care decisions.

Responsibilities among welfare workers are complex within the fragmented service system (Clarke 2004; Möttönen and Kettunen 2014). Hence, it is likely that professional responsibilities may be differently defined and understood, resulting in negotiations between the different stakeholders. The notion of boundaries is useful in studying the division of responsibilities because it focuses on how social actors construct groups as similar and different and how boundaries shape their understanding of responsibilities (Lamont and Molnár 2002). In other words, as workers discuss their responsibilities, they come to define their own scope of practice in relation to those of others, and to set boundaries between "our" tasks and expertise and those of "others". For example, Atkinson (2004) notes how physicians discursively construct their and "others'" competence and responsibility in medical collegial talk.

We begin by discussing welfare workers' boundary negotiations in relation to risk management, and their status as grass-roots level workers within a multi-professional field of community care. Following this, we introduce and develop boundary work as a frame for the analysis. By analysing welfare workers' collegial talk in team meetings, we focus on the ways they negotiate and justify the boundaries of their responsibilities in relation to those of collaborating workers from other organisations. The analysis concentrates on those instances of talk where welfare workers discuss their clients' situations that are changing in some ways, and thus promotes talk about the responsibilities and possible risks involved.

Risk management in the core of boundary negotiations

The notion of risk is inherent in current welfare policies that are particularly inclined to "the questions of future predictability and controllability" (Borosch *et al.* 2016; Harrikari *et al.* 2014: 5). In particular, community care in England is identified as having a strong focus on risk management (Godin 2004; Joyce 2001; Stepney and Popple 2008), while the Finnish implementation of risk management is noted to be more moderate (Koskiaho 2014). However, policies in both countries pinpoint the gaps between services as notable risks that need to be prevented by more fluent collaboration between services (Schneider *et al.* 1999; World Health Organisation 2010). Thus collaboration as a means to manage risk in the fragmented service system can be seen to require increasing boundary negotiations among workers.

According to Kemshall *et al.* (1997), the responsibilities for managing risks are being relocated from the state to the delegated organisations in community care, which includes the margins of welfare services. The result of the relocation of risk management in the grass-roots level of community care is that workers have to adopt their own organisational processes of risk management (Kemshall *et al.* 1997). The same has happened in various professional fields, where professionals are assumed to manage the increasing uncertainty and anxiety of a complex "risk society" (Beck 1992; Fenwick 2016: 57). Risk management has become a professional responsibility where each individual worker is obliged to calculate risks as central to their professional conduct (Joyce 2001; Miller and Rose 2008: 107–108). Welfare workers are extensively engaged with the issues of risks in their daily practices (Chapters 2 and 7; Parton 1996: 98; Godin 2004; Sawyer *et al.* 2009). Some risks relate more clearly to workers' own professional position. In these cases, risk management is seen to ensure workers' personal safety and to fulfil their accountability requirements from their organisation's perspective (Godin 2004: 355; Sawyer *et al.* 2009: 367, 371).

Besides their professional position, workers are primarily expected to enable their clients to deal with several risks (Evetts 2003). These include the risks that clients might pose to themselves (Godin 2004) or those that they might pose to other people or wider society (Miller and Rose 2008: 107). Thus, workers are responsible for the advice that they give and the success of the interventions that they carry out to manage the risk (Miller and Rose 2008: 107). Risk management is at the core of what Brodwin (2013: 68, 69) sees as mental health workers' responsibilities: ensuring stability in clients' lives by keeping the client safe, within housing and out of institutions. In other words, as "agents of stability" (Brodwin 2013: 66), workers are responsible for preventing crises in regard to psychiatric problems, residence or social relationships. Risks arise especially when changes of some sort take place in the client's life, such as when they are transferred to another service or their well-being is deteriorating. As noted in Chapter 2, within these situations, workers are held responsible in assessing the risks in terms of "high-risk" situations – for example, when a client evaluated as suicidal returns home from hospital. Workers are also responsible for "small-scale" risks, such as a client missing a doctor's appointment if not reminded by the professionals.

Both high and small-scale risks trigger boundary negotiations among workers, as we will see in the empirical section. Negotiations on professional boundaries are carried out regarding questions such as the following. What is the best way to handle and respond to the changes in the client's life? Who will do what? Who has the competence to make recommendations and decisions? This need for workers to carry out constant negotiations on risks is in accordance with what Broadhurst *et al.* (2010: 1047) call "informal logics of everyday risk management". The welfare workers' team meetings are one important arena for these mundane negotiations, and are studied in this chapter.

Shifting professional boundaries in community care

There has been a widespread fragmentation of services in social and health care (Clarke 2004; Evans 2010; Möttönen and Kettunen 2014). In Finland, community care has traditionally been conducted by non-governmental organisations (Koskiaho 2014), while the recent developments in health and social care policies have brought private companies into the field (Tynkkynen *et al.* 2013; Chapter 10 of this volume). In the UK, around two-thirds of the social care workforce is outside the public sector (Kessler and Bach 2011: 86). In community care in particular, workers are employed by multiple state and non-state agencies (Scourfield 2015: 928) such as private companies and public and semi-public service providers, as well as non-profit associations.

At the grass-roots level of community care, professional boundaries are shifting as a response to an increased diversity of professional and voluntary stakeholders in the field. The boundaries of professional responsibilities have partly been blurred by the transition from hospital-based interventions to community care (Brown *et al.* 2000), where workers have various educational backgrounds and collaborate beyond the boundaries of their own occupational group and organisation (Chong *et al.* 2013; Mossberg 2013). The multiplicity of community care requires effective interaction skills from workers to successfully negotiate the responsibilities with others. At the same time, clients' life spheres and the range of challenges they face are widening, requiring welfare workers to employ an almost all-encompassing orientation that takes into account the complexity of clients' situations (Brodwin 2013). In this context, the issue of boundaries becomes problematic in two ways: first, the functioning of welfare services is not limited to a single location, but is dispersed around several organisations; and second, collaboration between inter-professional teams is noted to lack formal and mutually shared boundary structures (Brown *et al.* 2000). These issues relate to wider shifts taking place within inter-professional boundaries, and the nature of the work undertaken by different health and social care professionals (Hopkins *et al.* 1996; Nancarrow and Borthwick 2005).

One motivation for shifting boundaries among welfare workers can be traced to managerial systems and practices that have been developed to constrain the autonomy of public service workers and to regulate their activities; not just measuring their performances, but reorganising the whole basis of service provision. While there is much debate about what constitutes the defining characteristics of a profession (Laffin and Entwistle 2000) and the extent of managerial surveillance, the contested status of workers in public services can be seen as being less about traits and more about relational characteristics. As Noordegraaf (2007: 774–775) puts it, "this calls for interdisciplinary knowledge and interactive skills. Professionals know how to operate in organized, interdisciplinary settings that cannot be organized easily; they know that cases, clients, costs and capacities are interrelated." Noordegraaf calls such workers "hybrid professionals". They are flexible, able to move around systems, to adapt to changing environments and search for occupational identities. One example of workers' ability to cross boundaries is the flexibility with which they move between social and health issues, thus operating as "hybrid sociomedical workers" (Brodwin 2013: 56). In addition to employing both social and health orientations with their clients, welfare workers can be characterised as "hybrid" in the sense that besides mastering the contents of client work, they know how to portray their work as efficient for managers (Saario 2014). Likewise, hybrid medical professionals are found to possess management accounting expertise in addition to their more traditional clinical skills (Kurunmäki 2004).

Social workers are pivotal collaborators with welfare workers. In the development of community care, the social work role in adult services has taken on a pivotal role, particularly in England. As the state is less of a provider of services, and commissions services from others, it is the social worker who is responsible for assessing need, purchasing services and managing packages of care, or as Malin (2000: 12) says, acting as "a broker". In some municipalities, the name has changed from "social worker" to "care manager". Lymbury (2000: 134) considers that the key boundary issue is the effect on the social worker's relationship with the client. He considers them to have taken on largely technical responsibilities, with the centrality of developing an in-depth relationship with the client having been reduced. Indeed, the social worker–client relationship is "unnecessary, even distracting", as the key task is gathering information "to make a categorization on which a subsequent purchase is made" (Lymbury 2000: 134). Also, in Finland, the role of a social worker is noted to be increasingly that of a designer, manager and coordinator of service processes, whereas less educated social and health care workers conduct the actual face-to-face community care work with clients (Sarvimäki and Siltaniemi 2007: 40–42).

Community care is noted to signify new territories for paramedical and associated professions, such as welfare workers who are able to colonise new spaces to operate in – for example, home visiting (Prior 1993). Thus the retreat of the social worker from the caring role has opened a space for welfare workers as providers of care and support. Malin (2000: 15) highlights the influential Griffiths Report (1988: para. 8.4), which suggested the creation of "a community carer" to undertake "the front-line personal and social support of dependent people". Such workers should provide "assistance required without demarcation problems arising". In other words, they should be flexible and not bound to professional allegiances. The number of welfare workers, such as care workers and support assistants, has increased significantly over the last 15 years (Kessler *et al.* 2006); they are often under the direction of more highly educated staff (Nancarrow *et al.* 2005).

While housing support workers have been employed by municipalities (and housing associations in England) to enable vulnerable clients to maintain their tenancy, the extension of support for clients with special needs is relatively new. As discussed above, the housing support worker has characteristics similar to assistant roles created in the community care policies. They visit clients regularly in their homes (between one and three times a week), and work to support plans covering everyday tasks concerned with health, employment, recreation, medication, personal and social skills, notable budgeting and tenancy maintenance. As Cameron (2010: 102) notes, it is "a role which previously might have been provided by a social worker or probation office". An essential part of these tasks is managing the risks involved and assessing who is responsible in which situation.

Analysing workers' negotiations on boundaries

Due to welfare workers' grass-roots position in community care, their involvement in risk management is essential to study from the point of view of professional boundaries. Focusing on workers' team meetings, the empirical analysis examines especially how workers in non-governmental mental health organisations define their responsibilities in relation to other professionals in the field. Most workers have vocational qualifications in social and health care, while some have undergone training with no degree. They work for two services. The first is an English floating support service for people with mental health problems; the workers collaborate mostly with their clients' care coordinators and services providing home care or medical assistance. The second is a Finnish project offering housing and social skills training for young adults with diagnosed schizophrenia; the workers collaborate mainly with psychiatric outpatient clinics, social services, and other supported housing and daytime activity schemes. As inter-professional and inter-agency collaboration is an essential part of the work, the services are ideal contexts for studying the boundaries of different responsibilities. Further demands for collaboration are set by their "half way nature": services provide support only on a relatively short-term basis (from a few months to a maximum of around two years) and thus deal with frequent client transitions where they collaborate both with the services from where the clients are coming and those to where the clients are heading.

Boundary work is closely intertwined with professional responsibilities – for example, Allen (2000) considers boundary work to entail negotiations on the division of responsibilities. Boundary work involves a demarcation between insiders and outsiders (Lamont and Molnár 2002). From an interactional and discursive perspective, Juhila and Hall (Chapter 4) describe boundary work as a situated practice where professional and organisational demarcation is carried out, including (re)negotiations of responsibilities. In a similar vein, Slembrouck and Hall (2014: 62) refer to boundary work as the ways in which workers and clients manage "the dilemmas of the personal, professional, organisational and cultural divisions during everyday encounters". In this chapter, we concentrate on the accomplishments of boundary work where workers differentiate themselves from others on the basis of their particular responsibilities. These can be termed as discourses of competence which are tied to the evaluation of others' and the speaker's own knowledge, opinions and actions (Atkinson 2004: 13).

As a regular part of professional work, team meetings are ordinary everyday practices where workers' talk can be analysed from an ethnomethodological perspective (Garfinkel 1967). Viewed as interaction of a group of workers with more-or-less equal tasks, meetings can be analysed as joint negotiation on the responsibilities of the team members and of those outside the team. We approach the negotiation of responsibilities as a process by which boundaries, demarcations or other divisions are constructed (Wikström 2008: 60). A useful analytical concept for this approach is boundary work, which was introduced originally by Thomas Gieryn (1983). Boundary work frames our analysis by recognising talk on boundaries as discursive negotiations, as pointed out by Riesch (2010). There is always a goal in boundary work; in this case, to sort out the responsibilities.

When analysing workers' negotiations as boundary work, we look at the ways they produce justifications for workers' own and other's responsibilities. Justifications are accounts or statements given "to explain unanticipated or untoward behavior" and to neutralise the behaviour or action and its consequences (Scott and Lyman 1968: 46, 51). We aim to use justification to demonstrate a two-fold construction of boundaries. First, workers delegate responsibility to others, with the rationale "this does not belong to us since it demands other kinds of skills than ours". In other words, they exclude responsibilities that do not belong to them. This is called "exclusionary boundary work" in Chapter 4. Second, assuming more responsibility for workers themselves draws on the notion that "this belongs to our domain of work because we have the skills, thus we are the ones that can best support the client". In Chapter 4, this is called "inclusionary boundary work". In the analysis, we view inclusiveness and exclusiveness from the workers' perspective, i.e. how they jointly talk about excluding or including themselves in particular situations of clients — not how they exclude or include others.

Team meetings are occasions for workers to carry out collegial talk by discussing the latest developments of the clients within the current caseload. Furthermore, the meetings enable the planning of subsequent interventions. The familiarity of team meetings makes them particularly important occasions for boundary construction, as workers can freely address and even question the boundaries between theirs and others' responsibilities and forms of expertise. The informality of team meetings is partly due to their "backstage" nature with no audience (Goffman 1990). Questioning the expertise of others would probably not appear "at the front stage", i.e. wider meetings with outsiders – such as managers, collaborators or clients. The meetings can be described as arenas for informal talk that allow straightforward conversations and upfront descriptions about absent parties, such as clients (Juhila *et al.* 2014a: 166; Urek 2005) or workers from other agencies (Saario *et al.* 2015).

In the forthcoming analyses, we present four examples of floating support and project workers' joint negotiation on boundaries of responsibilities. Each example features a particular responsibility:

1   the responsibility for maintaining contact with the client;
2   the responsibility for maintaining an adequate level of support;
3   the responsibility for safeguarding the client's future;
4   the responsibility for informing one's own professional view for collaborators.

In each example, workers discuss a case where a change is currently taking place in the client's life. We assume that changes in the client's situation promote talk about responsibilities and possible risks more often than stable situations (see also Scott 1997). We pay special attention to how the boundaries of responsibilities are justified and negotiated among workers concerning specific client cases.

Exclusionary and inclusionary boundary work

Negotiating boundaries of responsibilities when maintaining contact with the client

The first team meeting extract is from a floating support service in England. The client discussed in this example is a woman in her thirties who is visited at home by the floating support (FS) workers three times a week. Her well-being is acutely challenged due to her hearing voices and her refusal to let the workers into her home. In the meeting, maintaining contact with the client in this changed situation arises as the key professional responsibility.

In this extract, FS workers bring up two other parties with whom they collaborate. First is the Crisis team that specialises in clients with urgent and severe mental health problems. They usually become involved when intensified and specialised psychiatric home treatment is required. Second is the client's care coordinator from the local psychiatric outpatient clinic, who is a community psychiatric nurse (CPN). FS workers are in a regular contact with the CPN regarding the client's care plan and overall situation, especially now that these problems have arisen. Worker 1, who is chairing the meeting, initiates the discussion on the client by stating her initials.

Extract 1.1

1 WORKER 1: WM.
2 WORKER 2: A bit of a crisis on Tuesday with her. I rang her about her review, she was supposed to have her review on Tuesday, and she was screaming down the phone, tried to speak to her and she wouldn't communicate with me at all. Rang Crisis, they didn't want to know because it was nearly 9 o'clock. Spoke to her CPN, and we went out at 10 o'clock and she's shaved all her hair off, her eyebrows off, wouldn't speak to us, was writing stuff down for us saying that a male voice wouldn't let her talk. But he [the male voice delusion that the client hears in her head] spoke to us saying that he didn't want to harm her, he just wanted to make her suffer. CPN rang Crisis and they said that we were fine to leave her because her voice said that she was going to be safe, because it wasn't going to hurt her. Crisis went out and seen her Wednesday morning, then she refused to let them in Wednesday afternoon, they wouldn't have any contact with her. And then they went back out yesterday morning and she let them in, but she's still not talking. I've tried contacting her myself a couple of times during the week, but it seems that she's unplugged her phone from the wall, so I can't get through to her.

Worker 2 starts describing the intensified and changed situation of the client by reporting a phone call with the client, who would not communicate with her. She uses the client's unwillingness to speak to her as a justification for consequent requests for other professionals to come on board. First, she called Crisis, which declined the request on the basis of the time of the call: in office hours, the primary professional to be contacted is the care coordinator. Here, exclusionary boundary work takes place, as the responsibility for maintaining contact with the client is directed to workers of other organisations than floating support.

After speaking to the CPN, worker 2 visited the client together with the CPN, suggesting that worker 2 does not completely exclude herself from this responsibility but rather shares it, although we do not know how far the CPN or support worker directs this visit. Worker 2 then reports her observations from the home visit to indicate the severity of the situation: the client has shaved her hair off and hears a voice that forbids her to talk to the workers, so the client communicates with the workers in writing. At the site, the CPN contacts Crisis and receives permission for herself and worker 2 "*to leave*" the client. Crisis is heard to justify such an assessment as the client's voice indicates that she "*is going to be safe*" which is considered to indicate that she would not hurt herself. So Crisis is portrayed as the agency responsible for the consecutive home visits and for maintaining contact with the client, as is justified by the severity of the situation.

In the last sentence, worker 2 assumes some responsibility back by reporting that she has been trying to contact the client by phone, albeit without response. The phone calls were carried out despite Crisis being responsible for maintaining contact with the client. The calls can be interpreted as a caring attitude and concern of FS workers towards the client. By trying to reach the client "voluntarily", FS workers are doing an extra bit beyond their current responsibility, which can be interpreted as an attempt to justify their role with the client as still being important even though others have assumed responsibility for decision-making. The meeting continues with the dialogue between the two previous speakers and worker 3:

Extract 1.2

  3   WORKER 1: Right.
  4   WORKER 2: But Crisis are dealing with it and they're going to let us know.
  5   WORKER 1: What do you think is usually the outcome of this kind of thing –
        is it, like, admittance to hospital or ...
  6   WORKER 2: It depends.
  7   WORKER 1: Right.
  8   WORKER 2: We've got to wait to see what Crisis do; it's up to them to make
        the decision, not us.
  9   WORKER 1: And they're getting in touch with us when they're ...
 10   WORKER 2: They'll get in touch with [the CPN] who should be getting in
        touch with me.
 11   WORKER 1: Right.
 12   WORKER 2: Which is what's been agreed, but ...
 13   WORKER 1: If that doesn't work out, obviously just give them a call.
 14   WORKER 2: I ring them every day anyway.
 15   WORKER 1: OK, that's all right then. Not much we can do if it's like that.
 16   WORKER 2: There isn't anything we can do, just keep trying to contact her.
 17   WORKER 1: OK. It's not worth going out, is it?
 18   WORKER 3: No.
 19   WORKER 2: No, we're not allowed to.
 20   WORKER 3: We're not allowed to when she's unwell, because of previous
        risks.
 21   WORKER 1: Obviously that's Crisis's job.
 22   WORKER 2: Yeah, because her voice wanted to kill me before.
 23   WORKER 1: Right, well, that's fair enough.

This extract continues to demonstrate joint accomplishment of exclusionary boundary work, on the basis of which FS workers terminate their home visits for now. The responsibility for maintaining contact with the client is justified by the active involvement of Crisis, who are now "*dealing with it*" and "*going to let us know*", as worker 2 says (turn 4) after being affirmed by the chair. Thus the FS service is positioned as awaiting contact from Crisis. In turn 5, the chair introduces another possible intervention besides home visiting, and asks others' opinion regarding the likelihood of the client's admission to a psychiatric hospital. Worker 2 sees this also as Crisis's duty: "*it's up to them to make the decision, not us*" (turn 8). The chair confirms this by saying that Crisis will inform them; worker 2 specifies in more detail that FS workers will hear from Crisis through the CPN, "*who should be getting in touch with me*", thus delineating a longer chain of responsibility. Worker 2 uses the formulation "*should*", which might imply a slight uncertainty about whether this will happen. The uncertainty becomes obvious also in turn 12, where worker 2 displays the current state of affairs (without anyone asking): "*Which is what's been agreed but ...*"; this also repeats the justification for exclusionary boundary work of FS workers. In turn 13, the chair takes back some responsibility by giving advice on how to proceed: if they do not hear from the CPN, they will call her. The chair is extending FS workers' responsibility from the previous position, where they would merely await contact from others. If the CPN does not fulfil her responsibility for contacting the floating support, FS workers will contact her on their own initiative: "*obviously just give them a call*", by which they might want to make sure that the CPN handles the situation as agreed or that they are not excluded from future decisions. Worker 2, however, neutralises this into ordinary action by stating that she calls them "*every day anyway*". In turn 16, worker 2 demonstrates FS workers' simultaneous exclusion and inclusion from their responsibilities, which are inconsistent: "*There isn't anything we can do, just keep trying to contact her.*" In summary, the negotiated boundaries can be characterised as mainly exclusionary, as this indicates a narrower responsibility compared with FS workers' usual responsibility for carrying out regular home visits.

From turn 17 onwards, exclusionary boundary work is accomplished again and is now justified by risk. The workers jointly narrow their responsibility of "*going out*" to meet the client because of the concern for their own safety. In turn 20, worker 3 relates the risk to organisational risk aversion guidelines: FS workers "*are not allowed*" to do home visits "*because of previous risks*", thus indicating an external procedural constraint on possible action. They may face sanction from their own organisation if they attempt a home visit in such circumstances. The chair confirms once again that contacting the client is "*obviously ... Crisis's job*". Worker 2 agrees and specifies the type of risk on the basis of her history with the client: there has been an incident where the client's voice threatened to kill her. In the light of this risk, home visiting is not even an option for FS workers. This echoes the findings of Sawyer *et al.* (2009: 367) on mental health workers following risk management procedures, both to ensure their own security and to fulfil accountability requirements from their organisation's perspective.

Extracts 1.1. and 1.2. can be described as "action-oriented boundary work" (see Slembrouck and Hall 2014: 70), where maintaining contact with the client is recognised as a responsibility that must be fulfilled by doing something, often resulting in negotiations on who will do it – FS workers or someone else. The workers repeatedly use verbs that indicate the responsibility of other services. They exclude themselves from this responsibility, as well as from the decision on whether to start preparing the possible hospital admission. However, the exclusion is justified by them having passed on concerns appropriately to other, specialist professionals, as they can now be assured that the client is being taken care of.

Negotiating boundaries of responsibilities when maintaining adequate support

In the next extract, a change has taken place when the client returns home after being discharged from the psychiatric hospital. The situation is the opposite of the previous example in the sense that here the client, a woman in her forties, is getting better and her delusions have dramatically reduced. The workers are from the same English floating support service, and are now negotiating responsibilities that concern providing an adequate amount of support. Boundaries of responsibilities are negotiated between the CPN's office, the psychiatric hospital, the home care and the supported housing unit / floating support service. Worker 1, who is chairing the team meeting, initiates the discussion by stating the client's initials and telling the other workers about the client's CPA meeting.

Extract 2

1   WORKER 1: PM. We attended, [Worker 3] and I attended the CPA last week. It was noted that her delusions had dramatically reduced. She was getting loads better, wasn't she, basically, was what they said?

2   WORKER 2: Yeah.

3   WORKER 1: She's not as unwell. She was going on home leave for that weekend, and had [domiciliary service], was it?

4   WORKER 2: Yeah.

5   WORKER 1: Going in four times a day, and Crisis team, was it, that were going in as well over the weekend, to make sure she was coping OK at home. Providing everything went well, which I'm assuming it did, she is being discharged from [psychiatric hospital] today. It was said that we [floating support] will still attend for one hour a week on a Friday, but we don't feel that's enough. I think I said this to you last week, didn't I, an hour is not enough? So we need to kind of get in contact with …

6   WORKER 2: [care coordinator].

7   WORKER 3: Who?

8   WORKER 1: [care coordinator].

9   WORKER 2: Or [substitute for the care coordinator].

10   WORKER 3: Yeah.

11   WORKER 1: Yeah, to kind of up her hours and give her two hours back.

12   WORKER 3: Two hours' support a week.
13   WORKER 1: Because an hour's not long enough, so we need to try and get another hour put in place, so she can have the two hours on the Friday. She's on quite a high dose of ... I never remember medication.
14   WORKER 2: Quetiapine?
15   WORKER 1: Quetiapine, that's the one, she's on quite a high dose of that, but I think home care are going to be dealing with all that, aren't they? They said they were going in quite a lot, so.... And basically ours is just community access.
16   WORKER 2: Yeah, getting her out and about, yeah.

In turns 1–5, the workers report previous developments with the client, how other professionals have been involved and how they have evaluated the clients' improved condition. Consequently, the client was discharged from the hospital. At the end of turn 5, worker 1 continues to report how others had made a decision and what *"was said"* about their role in the client's care: *"we [floating support] will still attend for one hour a week on a Friday"*. She does not accept this, believing they should be more involved. The workers are promoting their role and importance in this case by contacting the care coordinator and trying to get back two hours' support for the client, which had been the case before. The workers' talk reflects the inclusionary boundary work, as they need to be more involved. Nevertheless, they are not explicitly explaining why they need to get that one hour back, except that two hours was the amount of hours before the hospital period. In turns 13–16, the workers note the high dose of medicine the client is taking, and exclude themselves from dealing with it, as it falls under the home care's responsibility. The increased amount of floating support might be implicitly justified by the high dose of medication: although worker 1 does not directly connect these two, she first states that the client *"can have two hours on the Friday"* and continues by noting the high dose of medication. As such a high dose is needed, the client also requires her hours to be doubled, to allow for FS workers *"getting her out and about"*. The high dose of medicine might indicate the risk of the client remaining isolated in her home.

This extract from the team meeting demonstrates mostly inclusionary boundary work, as the workers conclude that they need to include themselves more in the client's case than has been proposed by the others. This example represents action-oriented boundary work (Slembrouck and Hall 2014), as there is talk about who should do certain things (take care of medication), but also authority-oriented boundary work, as there are negotiations about who has the authority to decide their contribution to the client's care in the future. By "authority-oriented" boundary work we refer to negotiations on who has the right to decide and whose professional opinion is taken seriously by others, thus differing from action-oriented boundary work on who will do what (see Slembrouck and Hall 2014). In the end part, the boundaries are more negotiable and exclusionary (medicine taking) in relation to their expertise. All in all, the extract demonstrates the functioning of a home visit as a key vehicle for monitoring risk

(Broadhurst *et al.* 2010). The responsibilities for managing the risk of isolation are negotiated by considering both social and medical issues – in other words, by employing "hybrid orientation".

Negotiating boundaries of responsibilities when safeguarding the client's future

In the third extract, we present meeting talk about the client, a man in his early thirties who is currently living in the Finnish project that offers supported housing and social skills training for young adults with diagnosed schizophrenia. The major change around which the discussion revolves is the client's upcoming transition as the project is ending, and there is a need to find alternative supported accommodation. The project workers' task is to evaluate the options for supported housing or floating support based on the assessment they make during the project. Instead of an official decision, they only make recommendations for the formal decision-making carried out by the commissioner and the psychiatrist in charge. The key responsibilities discussed concern communicating the current status of the client's ill-health and mundane living skills so that other professionals can safeguard his future. There are four project workers in this particular meeting, but in this extract, three of these are talking about arranging a network meeting for the client. Worker 1 comments on the idea of inviting the home rehabilitation team to the meeting.

Extract 3

1   WORKER 1: I think we probably should ask them [floating support], because we are a bit, when we were talking they didn't actually have a clue that [client] even had these terrible delusions.

2   WORKER 2: I was just thinking the same when [worker of floating support] popped in there, to ask something, she just said that, oh he was such a funny guy, this [client].

3   WORKER 3: Yeah, a lovely guy with such good stories to tell.

4   WORKER 2: And also [another worker of home rehabilitation team] – I was there just for a little while, but anyhow, when [worker from the project] said that we have thought that it is really hard for [client] to live independently, well, [worker of home rehabilitation team mentioned above] was genuinely surprised by that – like, really, why would you think that?

5   WORKER 1: No way, oh my goodness! Really, that's horrible.

6   WORKER 2: There's the thing as well that before [client] has used his car to get to places, but now he has realised himself that he doesn't really, like, there's stuff, like, he cannot drive on – bridges, for example – and now he has understood to leave the car completely.

[Removed: talking about the past when the client was still driving]

7   WORKER 1: Well, this really must be initiated, I think, bit by bit. Now he has all the necessary information, at least regarding how to live at home and

how, how important it is to have a kind of regular rhythm so that it doesn't go to that, and then all these arrangements and controls and visits – but, we'll see it in the follow-up period, that, whether this works or not, and then I think we should collaborate with these, you know, these ...

8   WORKER 2: We could ask the home rehabilitation team.

9   WORKER 1: The home rehabilitation team and, these people, [client's nurse from the psychiatric outpatient clinic], or what was the name?

10   WORKER 2: Would they come then, and the home team ladies [refers to home rehabilitation team], and possibly the GP into the same meeting, where we could state the situation, what we think is going on? And then we have, in my opinion, kind of transferred this bit to them. You know all these things like measuring blood sugar levels and all, I mean, if he will be having insulin, so someone should visit there, home-based nursing services to give that medicine to him. Plus that pill dispenser, it's in a right state, oh my god!

[Overlapping speech]

11   WORKER 1: Yeah, both the care of the psyche and the physics, it all depends on [client] really – well, that cannot work out like that.

[Removed: discussing available dates for the network meeting]

12   WORKER 1: Yep. We could offer a date [for the meeting], because apparently it seems unclear for quite many [people], for example the psychological condition of his, that, how much he has these delusions and fears in the end.

In the beginning, worker 1 justifies the need to involve the rehabilitation team in the network meeting with other collaborators who she poses as lacking relevant, up-to-date knowledge about the client: "*they didn't actually have a clue that [he] even had these terrible delusions*". Then workers 2 and 3 confirm this by using reported speech (Holt and Clift 2007) of another worker, which also demonstrates that the collaborator is not up to date with the seriousness of the client's condition. In turn 4, there is a reference to yet another worker, who has the same kind of misunderstanding and lack of knowledge about the situation: "*[worker] was genuinely surprised by that – like, really, why would you think that?*" There is also a reference to their colleague's evidence of the client's difficulties in living independently. Then worker 1 assesses the situation with criticism and upgraded terms: "*No way, oh my goodness! Really, that's horrible,*" which is evidence of backstage talk shared by "insiders" (Goffman 1990). Thus, the project workers separate their competence from that of other collaborators, as they are holding the "everyday evidence" (Saario *et al.* 2015) of a client, while collaborators are presented as lacking this knowledge. Inclusionary boundary work is based on everyday evidence to influence the decision on the most appropriate living arrangement for the client (see also Scourfield 2015).

In turn 6, worker 2 describes how they are up to date on the seriousness of the client's situation and have clear evidence that the client is not capable of certain things, such as driving. Here, worker 2 establishes the client's incapability of driving as a fact based on evidence that is outside the worker's own subjective assessment. The establishment of factual evidence (Smith 1978) is strengthened by the positive side that also the client himself has realised this problem. Thus, worker 2 justifies their everyday evidence by encouraging collaborators to see the seriousness of the situation. In turn 7, worker 1 describes how they have succeeded in rehabilitating the client, and with this she also justifies the exclusionary boundary work: we've performed our responsibility to train the client regarding everyday skills, and we will follow up on this. This is confirmed in turns 8 and 9: the exclusion will be actualised by inviting the home rehabilitation team and psychiatric nurse to the network meeting. Overall, the workers' talk replicates the need to update other collaborators regarding the serious mental ill-health of the client. In that sense, they need to be included alongside other collaborators.

In turns 10 and 12, worker 2 summarises the possible future participants in the network meeting. Thus, her talk reflects the exclusionary boundary work, as they are handing the overall responsibility to the outpatient clinic, another floating support service and the GP. It also includes a suggestion to recruit a new service – a home-based nursing service – as there is a need for health care expertise with the medication and measuring of blood sugars. In turn 10, worker 2 furthermore justifies the exclusionary boundary work, as the network meeting needs to be organised so that other parties can be brought up to date regarding the client's serious mental ill-health.

This team meeting talk is interesting as it demonstrates different justifications for boundary work from the previous example. Here inclusionary boundary work is justified by others not being up to date on the client's condition and ill-health. Now, as the client is leaving the service, workers need to include other workers and also themselves in the network meeting in order to transfer the everyday evidence (helplessness, ill-health and need for support) to other collaborators. They want to ensure that their ways of thinking are adopted by other collaborators, so that in the future their assessments of the client's problems will remain definitive. By doing this, they are managing the possible risks regarding the client's situation in the transition process. The risk assessment and inclusionary boundary work are needed to communicate the situation in order to transfer the client properly and with enough support. Knowing the "client's best interests" also functions as a justification for inclusionary boundary work. This extract represents authority-oriented boundary work, as it is associated with assessing who has the most relevant knowledge and competence on the client, to be used as the basis of the decision on future support.

Negotiating boundaries of responsibilities when informing collaborators of workers' opinion

Our last extract is from the same Finnish project as Extract 3. The client is a young man in his early twenties. He has a history of several stays at the psychiatric hospital prior to the project. The responsibility to be negotiated concerns the communication of project workers' opinion to collaborators concerning the client's future support. Prior to this extract, the workers discuss the client continually changing his mind about where to live and what to study. Worker 4 (not talking in the extract) has said that the last time she talked to the client, he was not interested in moving to supported housing. In the previous turns, four project workers have been talking about the meeting that was held between the client, his parents, the municipal authorities and the social worker. In this extract they continue to talk about the meeting and wonder why they were not invited.

Extract 4

1   WORKER 1: I dunno how they'll [municipal authorities and the social worker] take this idea of [vocational training course], this Tuesday then, it's in bits and pieces, the whole thing with [client] is not being considered in a very client-centric manner, from their part. Money matters. The scariest thing is [client]'s well-being, that's how long will it take until his self-destructive thoughts arise again, although in the latest common meeting it was discussed, his self-destructiveness in general, that it's bad and poor and what's more, and [client] brought up himself that it has now improved while he has been [in the project], that he has gained self-confidence and cleared his own thoughts, he can now trust them [his thoughts] and doesn't have self-destructive thoughts. Well, we'll see how all this messing up affects him now.

2   WORKER 2: It would have been so important that someone from us would have attended that meeting where the social worker was, and ...

3   WORKER 1: That's right – why weren't we asked?

4   WORKER 2: Yeah exactly, well, our presence would have been very important, and especially as [client] is confronted with such high expectations, like you'll start studying and into the working life, plus all the hobbies on top of that.

5   WORKER 1: And independent living and ...

6   WORKER 3: I asked about this.

7   WORKER 2: So awful.

8   WORKER 1: Why weren't we asked, why wasn't [occupational therapist of project] or somebody invited? But somehow, what was the answer you got from [occupational therapist]?

9   WORKER 3: Well, as this is not, well not about [client] alone, but this is a kind of family counselling, so it is among them only and thus we don't go there, anyhow.

10 WORKER 1: We don't, we don't, but if they are having family counselling for this couple, well, why do they dig up all these [issues]?

11 WORKER 3: Yeah, my point exactly – that, why it has become all about discussing [client], this ...

12 WORKER 1: Yeah, [client] being in [this project].

In turn 1, worker 1 quite strongly evaluates other collaborators' (the municipal authorities' and the social worker's) involvement in this client's case as not being client-centric. Other collaborators' actions have caused concern that the client's condition may possibly get worse. Worker 1 justifies this by reporting the client's thoughts about his condition and how it was much improved in the project. The worker is wondering whether this is now threatened because of "*all this messing up*". Her/his talk implies quite a high risk of the client's situation getting worse and functions as justification for inclusionary boundary work: we have managed to support the client so that he is getting better; hence our views and involvement are essential in preventing the risks. Workers possess evidence of the client's improvements and, in their opinion, collaborators have set too-high expectations which negatively affect the client's well-being.

In subsequent turns, the workers are wondering why they were not invited to the meetings with social service authorities and thus not involved. They give justifications for inclusionary boundary work – their presence and involvement in the meetings would have been important, as other parties had set far too high expectations for the client. They report how they had asked why they were excluded from the meeting and what kind of answers they were given. In turns 10–12, the workers jointly justify the importance of their involvement, as they do not accept that the other parties would have talked about issues in the meeting that concerned them and their responsibility. The client's involvement in the project should not be on the agenda of such a meeting.

This extract represents mainly authority-oriented boundary work, as there is constant negotiation over who has the relevant knowledge and competence regarding the client and decisions to be made about his future. The workers' dialogue displays backstage talk (Goffman 1990) that enables them to criticise other collaborators and their judgements. This extract illustrates the risks related to overly fixed professional boundaries, as workers need to promote clients' well-being and at the same time they need to argue for their competence and the involvement of other collaborators. Hence, inclusionary boundary work is carried out to justify the team's further involvement in the client case.

Conclusion and discussion

Our discursive analysis supports the notion that boundaries are a pervasive feature of most professional practices and especially essential when professional responsibilities are negotiated (Allen 2000: 338–339; Hall *et al.* 2010: 349; Slembrouck and Hall 2014: 78). Boundaries are constructed in interaction (Hernes 2004) as workers communicate their specialities and restrictions to themselves and others. In team meetings, professional boundaries are mutually talked into being and negotiated in interaction, thus representing "a joint endeavor" of workers (Juhila *et al.* 2014a). For example, in the meetings the word "we" was frequently used instead of "I", and silent workers continually uttered affirmative words such as "yeah" to the speaker (these minimal responses were not transcribed in the extracts). Workers' team meetings can be seen as arenas for collective accountability, which indicates the sharing of responsibilities among the team members (Bell *et al.* 2011). To cite Lamont and Molnár (2002: 171), workers' collegial talk in team meetings reveals "with what kinds of inferences concerning similarities and differences groups mobilize to define who they are".

In this chapter, we presented four examples where workers are negotiating the boundaries of their responsibilities in situations where their clients are undergoing particular changes that indicate increased risk. The responsibilities include maintaining contact with the client and providing adequate support, safeguarding the client's future and informing collaborators about workers' up-to-date knowledge of the client case. By using boundary work as an analytical concept, we found that workers' and collaborators' responsibilities are talked into being by two distinct forms of boundary work: action-oriented and authority-oriented. Action-oriented boundary work (Slembrouck and Hall 2014) featured mostly in the first two examples, where workers negotiated boundaries for the provision of adequate support and maintaining contact with the client. Both were recognised as tasks that require action and specific interventions from the workers or their collaborators. Authority-oriented boundary work, on the other hand, was prevalent in the two last examples, on safeguarding the client's future and informing collaborators about the opinions of the workers. Workers mainly depicted others as not acting responsibly, while at the same time they justified themselves as experts in the clients' situations. Authority-oriented boundary work drew strongly on open criticism towards collaborators, to the extent that the meeting talk can be occasionally seen to include what Dingwall (1977) termed "atrocity stories".

In addition to authority and action orientations, boundary work also entails exclusionary or inclusionary dimensions that have ethical implications. This echoes with Slembrouck and Hall's (2014: 74) notion on boundary work having both enabling and constraining effects at the same time. Constraining issues relate to what we call exclusionary boundary work. This raises the question of whether the tightening of resources and the discourse of efficiency produce unwanted welfare service areas or client groups, which professions redefine out from their expertise. Although it is not evident in team meetings, exclusionary boundary work is important to analyse, as it might produce client groups that are not recognised as belonging to a specific expertise of any professions or organisations, or who are easily referred to other welfare organisations (Chapter 4). This points out the challenging situation of the margins of welfare services that are often places of last resort, where workers cannot draw strong boundaries regarding the client selection yet also need to include "difficult cases" in their caseload. Exclusionary boundary work is also used to responsibilise collaborators by delegating duties to them. Inclusionary boundary work, on the other hand, relates closely to the enabling effects of boundary work (Slembrouck and Hall 2014: 74), as it involves workers self-responsibilising themselves to take on more responsibilities and occasionally to go "the extra mile" (Doel *et al.* 2010). The workers construct themselves as a team drawing on the ethos of care and concern towards their clients. In both cases, responsibilisation is mainly carried out for the benefit of the client – for example, arranging the most suitable form of support. The way workers negotiate their boundaries reveals that their speciality lies within mundane observations based on their assessments of clients. By sharing everyday life with clients, they become familiar with their current well-being and needs, in contrast to collaborative professionals who see the client more rarely and are more distant.

In summary, the analysis of boundary work among welfare workers operating at the grass-roots level indicates a change in the division of labour in community care: to advocate their clients, welfare workers carry wide-ranging responsibilities towards them. Instead of limiting their professional interventions to everyday support, they engage in frequent negotiations to advocate and even coordinate the care of the clients. Furthermore, boundary work in changing client situations portrays risk management strongly as a negotiated activity (see also Allen 1997). Informal processes of shaping boundaries and related decisions, carried out in team meetings, pose a risk as an everyday issue that workers need to take into account, especially regarding the future of clients. In this light, risk management becomes understood more widely than as merely a set of standardised tools, such as "tick-box" forms or recording artefacts, that workers use to assess and manage risk (see Godin 2004; Juhila *et al.* 2014b). While formal tools are an effective way to display transparency of professional action, risk is eventually managed in face-to-face occasions within a relatively informal atmosphere – such as team meetings.

References

Allen, D. (1997) "The nursing-medical boundary: a negotiated order?", *Sociology of Health and Illness*, 19(4): 498–520.

Allen, D. (2000) "Doing occupational demarcation: the 'boundary work' of nurse managers in a district general hospital", *Journal of Contemporary Ethnography*, 29(3): 326–356.

Atkinson, P. (2004) "The discursive construction of competence and responsibility in medical collegial talk", *Communication & Medicine*, 1(1): 13–23.

Beck, U. (1992) *Risk Society: Towards a new modernity*, London: Sage.

Bell, S.K., Delbanco, T., Anderson-Shaw, L., McDonald, T. and Thomas, H.G. (2011) "Accountability for medical error: moving beyond blame to advocacy", *Chest Journal*, 140(2): 519–526.

Borosch, N., Kuhlmann, J. and Blum, S. (2016) "Opening up opportunities and risks? Retrenchment, activation and targeting as main trends of recent welfare state reforms across Europe", in K. Schubert, P. de Villota and J. Kuhlmann (eds) *Challenges to European Welfare Systems* (pp. 769–791), Cambridge: Springer International Publishing.

Broadhurst, K., Hall, C., Wastell, D., White, S. and Pithouse, A. (2010) "Risk, instrumentalism and the humane project in social work: identifying the informal logics of risk management in children's statutory services", *British Journal of Social Work*, 40(4): 1046–1064.

Brodwin, P.E. (2013) *Everyday Ethics: Voices from the frontline of community psychiatry*, Berkeley: University of California Press.

Brown, B., Crawford, P. and Darongkamas, J. (2000) "Blurred roles and permeable boundaries: the experience of multidisciplinary working in community mental health", *Health and Social Care in the Community*, 8(6): 425–435.

Cameron, A. (2010) "The contribution of housing support workers to joined-up services", *Journal of Interprofessional Care*, 24(1): 100–110.

Chong, W.W., Aslani, P. and Chen, T.F. (2013) "Shared decision-making and interprofessional collaboration in mental healthcare: a qualitative study exploring perceptions of barriers and facilitators", *Journal of Interprofessional Care*, 27(5): 373–379.

Clarke, J. (2004) "Dissolving the public realm? The logics and limits of neo-liberalism", *Journal of Social Policy*, 33(1): 77–101.

Dingwall, R. (1977) "'Atrocity stories' and professional relationships", *Work and Occupations*, 4(4): 371–396.

Doel, M., Allmark, P., Conway, P., Cowburn, M., Flynn, M., Nelson, P. and Tod, A. (2010) "Professional boundaries: crossing a line or entering the shadows?", *British Journal of Social Work*, 40(6): 1866–1889.

Evans, T. (2010) *Professional Discretion in Welfare Services: Beyond street-level bureaucracy*, Aldershot, UK: Ashgate.

Evetts, J. (2003) "The sociological analysis of professionalism: occupational change in the modern world", *International Sociology*, 18(2): 395–415.

Fenwick, T. (2016) *Professional Responsibility and Professionalism: A sociomaterial examination*, London: Routledge.

Garfinkel, H. (1967) *Studies in Ethnomethodology*, Cambridge: Polity Press.

Gieryn, T.F. (1983) "Boundary work and the demarcation of science from non-science: strains and interests in the professional ideologies of scientists", *American Sociological Review*, 48(6): 781–795.

Godin, P. (2004) "You don't tick boxes on a form: a study of how community mental health nurses assess and manage risk", *Health, Risk and Society*, 6(4): 347–360.

Goffman, E. (1990) *The Presentation of Self in Everyday Life*, London: Penguin Books.

Griffiths, R. (1988) *Community Care: An Agenda for Action*, London: HMSO.

Hall, C., Slembrouck, S., Haig, E. and Lee, A. (2010) "The management of professional and other roles during boundary work in child welfare", *International Journal of Social Welfare*, 19(3): 348–357.

Harrikari, T., Rauhala, P.-L. and Virokannas, E. (2014) "Modernization and social work: toward governing risks, advanced liberalism and crumbling solidarity?", in T. Harrikari, P.-L. Rauhala and E. Virokannas (eds) *Social Change and Social Work: The changing societal conditions of social work in time and place* (pp. 1–14), Surrey: Ashgate.

Hernes, T. (2004) "Studying composite boundaries: a framework of analysis", *Human Relations*, 57(1): 9–29.

Holt, E. and Clift, R. (eds) (2007) *Reporting Talk: Reported speech in interaction*. Cambridge: Cambridge University Press.

Hopkins, A., Solomon, J. and Abelson, J. (1996) "Shifting boundaries in professional care", *Journal of the Royal Society of Medicine*, 89(7): 364–371.

Håland, E. (2012) "Introducing the electronic patient record (EPR) in a hospital setting: boundary work and shifting constructions of professional identities", *Sociology of Health & Illness*, 34(5): 761–775.

Iqbal, N., Reese, M. and Backer, C. (2014) "Decision making, responsibility and accountability in community mental health teams", *Mental Health Practice*, 17(7): 26–28.

Joyce, P. (2001) "Governmentality and risk: setting priorities in the new NHS", *Sociology of Health & Illness*, 23(5): 594–614.

Juhila, K., Jokinen, A. and Saario, S. (2014a) "Reported speech", in C. Hall, K. Juhila, M. Matarese and C. van Nijnatten (eds) *Analysing Social Work Communication: Discourse in practice* (pp. 154–172), London: Routledge.

Juhila, K., Saario, S., Raitakari, S. and Gunther, K. (2014b) "Reported client-practitioner conversations as assessment in mental health", *Text & Talk*, 34(1): 69–88.

Kemshall, H., Parton, N. and Walsh, M. (1997) "Concepts of risk in relation to organizational structure and functioning within the personal social services and probation", *Social Policy and Administration*, 31(3): 213–232.

Kessler, I. and Bach, S. (2011) *The Modernisation of the Public Services and Employee Relations: Targeted change*, London: Palgrave Macmillan.

Kessler, I., Bach, S. and Heron, P. (2006) "Understanding assistant roles in social care", *Work Employment and Society*, 20(4): 667–685.

Koskiaho, B. (2014) *Kumppanuuden sosiaalipolitiikkaa etsimässä* [Searching for social policy of companionship], Helsinki: Setlementtiliitto.

Kurunmäki, L. (2004) "A hybrid profession: the acquisition of management accounting expertise by medical professionals", *Accounting, Organizations and Society*, 29(3–4): 327–347.

Laffin, M. and Entwistle, T. (2000) "New problems, old professions? The changing national world of the local government professions", *Policy and Politics*, 28(2); 207–220.

Lamont, M. and Molnár, V. (2002) "The study of boundaries in the social sciences", *Annual Review of Sociology*, 28(1): 167–195.

Lymbury, M. (2000) "The retreat from professionalism: from social worker to care manager", in N. Malin (ed.) *Professionalism, Boundaries and the Workplace* (pp. 123–138), London: Routledge.

Malin, N. (2000) "Professionalism and boundaries of the formal sector: the example of social and community care", in N. Malin (ed.) *Professionalism, Boundaries and the Workplace* (pp. 7–24), London: Routledge.

Miller, P. and Rose, N. (2008) *Governing the Present: Administering economic, social and personal life*, Cambridge: Polity Press.

Mossberg, L. (2013) "Strategic collaboration as means and ends: views from members of Swedish mental health strategic collaboration councils", *Journal of Interprofessional Care*, 28(1): 58–63.

Möttönen, S. and Kettunen, P. (2014) "Sosiaalipalvelut kuntien hallinto- ja palvelurakenteiden murroksessa" [Social services in the municipal administration and service structure reform], in R. Haverinen, M. Kuronen and T. Pösö (eds) *Sosiaalihuollon tila ja tulevaisuus* [The state and future of social welfare], Tampere: Vastapaino.

Nancarrow, S. and Borthwick, A. (2005) "Dynamic professional boundaries in the healthcare workforce", *Sociology of Health & Illness*, 27(7): 889–919.

Nancarrow, S., Shuttleworth, P., Tongue, A. and Brown, L. (2005) "Support workers in intermediate care", *Health and Social Care Community*, 13(4): 338–344.

Noordegraaf, M. (2007) "From 'pure' to 'hybrid' professionalism: present-day professionalism in ambiguous public domains", *Administration and Society*, 39(46): 761–785.

Parton, N. (1996) "Social work, risk and the 'blaming system'", in N. Parton (ed.) *Social Theory, Social Change and Social Work* (pp. 98–114), London: Routledge.

Prior, L. (1993) *The Social Organisation of Mental Illness*, London: Sage.

Riesch, H. (2010) "Theorizing boundary work as representation and identity", *Journal for the Theory of Social Behaviour*, 40(4): 452–473.

Saario, S. (2014) *Audit Techniques in Mental Health: Practitioners' responses to electronic health records and service purchasing agreements*, Tampere: Acta Universitatis Tamperensis, 1907.

Saario, S., Juhila, K. and Raitakari, S. (2015) "Boundary work in inter-agency and interprofessional client transitions", *Interprofessional Journal of Care*, 29(6): 610–615.

Sarvimäki, P. and Siltaniemi, A. (2007) *Recommendations for the Task Structure of Professional Social Services Staff*, Helsinki: Ministry of Social Affairs and Health, Finland.

Sawyer, A.-M., Moran, A. and Brett, J. (2009) "Should the nurse change the light globe? Human service professionals managing risk at the frontline", *Journal of Sociology*, 45(4): 361–381.

Schneider, J., Carpenter, J. and Brandon, T. (1999) "Operation and organisation of services for people with severe mental illness in the UK", *The British Journal of Psychiatry*, 175(5): 422–425.

Scott, D. (1997) "Inter-agency conflict: an ethnographic study", *Child and family social work*, 2(2): 73–80.

Scott, M. and Lyman, S. (1968) "Accounts", *American Sociological Review*, 33(1): 46–62.

Scourfield, P. (2015) "Even further beyond street-level bureaucracy: the dispersal of discretion exercised in decisions made in older people's care home reviews", *British Journal of Social Work*, 45(3): 914–931.

Slembrouck, S. and Hall, C. (2014) "Boundary work", in C. Hall, K. Juhila, M. Matarese and C. van Nijnatten (eds) *Analysing Social Work Communication: Discourse in practice* (pp. 61–78), London: Routledge.

Smith, D. (1978) "K is mentally ill: the anatomy of a factual account", *Sociology*, 23(12): 23–53.

Stepney, P. and Popple, K. (2008) *Social Work and the Community: A critical context for practice*, London: Palgrave Macmillan.

Tainio, L. and Wrede, S. (2008) "Practical nurses' work role and workplace ethos in an era of austerity", in S. Wrede, L. Henriksson, H. Høst, S. Johansson and B. Dybbroe (eds) *Care Work in Crisis: Reclaiming the Nordic ethos of care* (pp. 177–198), Lund, Sweden: Studenlitteratur.

Thompson, C. and Dowding, D. (2001) "Responding to uncertainty in nursing practice", *International Studies on Nursing Practice*, 38(5): 609–615.

Tynkkynen, L.-K., Keskimäki, I. and Lehto, J. (2013) "Purchaser–provider splits in health care: the case of Finland", *Health Policy*, 111(3): 221–225.

Urek, M. (2005) "Making a case in social work: the construction of an unsuitable mother", *Qualitative Social Work*, 4(4): 451–467.

Wikström, E. (2008) "Boundary work as inner and outer dialogue: dieticians in Sweden", *Qualitative Research in Organizations and Management: An International Journal*, 3(1): 59–77.

World Health Organisation (2010) *Framework for Action on Interprofessional Education & Collaborative Practice*, retrieved 18 May 2016 from www.who.int/hrh/resources/framework_action/en/.

10 Constructing service providers' responsibilities in interviews on commissioning

Sirpa Saario, Dorte Caswell and Christopher Hall

Introduction

Across Europe, various procedures and regulations are having a major impact on the management and organisation of service providers. Commissioning, including activities such as contracting and procurement, is one of the most crucial, having obligations to engage in competitive tendering in order to be contracted as providers. Furthermore, once providers secure a contract, various review systems are required to monitor and evaluate the outcomes of the services (Seymour 2010). Since 2000, relations between the state and the voluntary sector have increasingly been managed through market practices (Knapp *et al.* 2001; Cunningham and James 2009; Alcock 2010). Before this, the voluntary sector was based on principles of solidarity within civil society, often advocating for the rights of marginalised groups (Dufva 2005; Jordan and van Tuijl 2006). Along with commissioning, quasi-markets in social care (with competition amongst independent providers) have replaced monopoly provision by state bureaucracies (Vincent-Jones 2006: 180; Carmel and Harlock 2008; Bode *et al.* 2011). The basic principle is that the municipal authority will select "the providers who come closest to meeting its needs at the quality and quantity required and at an affordable price" (Wistow *et al.* 1992: 36).

Commissioning requires reformulating and specifying the differing responsibilities between commissioners and service providers (Stace and Cumming 2006; Rubery *et al.* 2012). This chapter investigates responsibilities of service providers, especially those that relate to their contractual duties within commissioning. We ask how the various responsibilities of non-governmental organisations (NGOs) acting as service providers are constructed, accounted for and resisted in the interview talk of the three parties: the managers of NGOs who provide the services, the commissioners who purchase the services, and the care coordinators who form a link between purchasers, providers and clients. Whereas commissioners and NGO managers have rather straightforward roles, the notion of the care coordinator might require explanation. As noted in Chapter 9, the care coordinator is a case manager, who is responsible for the client's care plan and managing the contribution of various service providers (Bayard *et al.* 1997; Onyett 1998). One care coordinator we interviewed explains her role as follows:

"I'm not there to provide that service. We're [care coordinators] coordinating that service to provide that support". Similarly, an interviewed manager of a service-providing organisation explains that the task of a care coordinator is to "put together a support plan. And then the project workers [of the service provider] basically deliver the support plans". However, the care coordinators studied in this chapter do not (as yet) control a budget to purchase services for their clients.

Initially, the chapter examines literature on commissioning in social and health services, to illustrate the responsibilities of service providers and the context in which they operate. The expectations towards providers within commissioning processes are then examined in the governmentality literature – more specifically, the ideas of contractual implication and the re-responsibilisation of providers are looked at. Furthermore, recovery as a welfare discourse is linked with the expectations that are set for providers. Empirical analysis draws on interviews with three key stakeholders in commissioning: commissioners, provider managers and care coordinators. Their talk regarding service providers' responsibilities is analysed by using the analytic concepts of accountability and resistance. Overall, the chapter demonstrates the responsibilities of providers to move their clients forward to more independent support, and the range of subtle ways to resist this responsibility.

Commissioning and purchaser–provider split

Commissioning is a feature of a market-based arrangement of organising social and health care, often according to the purchaser–provider model (Knapp *et al.* 2001; Tynkkynen *et al.* 2013). There is a split between municipal service purchasers and service providers, where the former commits to buy services under certain conditions, while the latter commits to provide them. In an external purchaser–provider model, the split between purchasers and providers is a particularly clear-cut one, because municipalities as purchasers do not provide any services themselves, but instead commission them exclusively from external providers – either private companies or NGOs (see Chapter 2). During recent decades, the funding based on tendering and contracts has significantly changed the role of providers, especially NGOs (Jordan and van Tuijl 2006; Vincent-Jones 2006; Chapter 2 of this volume). While NGOs have long histories in welfare services in Western welfare states, their role as external service providers is strikingly different from their previous status as charitable and voluntary organisations (e.g. Lundström and Svedberg 2003).

Public purchasing and procurement are subject to EU regulations (Sánchez Graells 2015). At the level of nation states, there are domestic contracting regimes. In England, the transition from bureaucratic to contractual organisation was initiated through policies of Compulsory Competitive Tendering (CCT). The NHS and Community Care Act (1990) introduced new institutional and organisational arrangements for the delivery of health, social and community care, including a purchaser–provider split. (Vincent-Jones 2006: 180–182.) In

Finland, the Public Procurement Act came into force in 2007 (Koskiaho 2008). The split between purchasers and competing providers was initially seen to lead to organisational flexibility and pluralism of service providers, instead of a monopoly of a few established providers (Tynkkynen *et al.* 2013). In both states, the pluralism (including both for-profit companies and NGOs) was expected to facilitate innovation and competition between providers to enhance choice and cost-effectiveness (Wistow *et al.* 1992; Tynkkynen *et al.* 2013). Tendering was recognised as the purest form of competition in a market where, ideally, all competitors have the same chance of obtaining a contract (Dyb and Loison 2007).

Contracting is an essential part of "the commissioning cycle" in which Rees (2014: 47–48; see also Bovaird *et al.* 2012) identifies four parts:

- the analysis of resources, providers and user needs;
- the planning of commissioning strategy and service design;
- procurement and delivery through tendering and contracting;
- monitoring and reviewing through contracting.

In contrast to previous grants to NGOs (Rees *et al.* 2014: 15), contracting is noted to become a significant organising principle for public reforms in general, and for social policy reforms in particular (Nilssen and Kildal 2009: 305), to the extent that it can now be regarded as the main medium of communication in the public sector. A contract is a legal document that sets out the expectations of the parties involved and defines their responsibilities. According to Lane (1999: 185), contracting involves "stipulating clear conditions about what has been agreed to: what is to be delivered; who is to pay; what additional obligations have been consented to?"

Contracting makes explicit responsibilities both to commissioners and providers, and affects their reciprocal relations (Rubery *et al.* 2012). As Tsui and Cheung (2004: 440) note: "Relationships are legal, time-limited, and task-oriented entities with clearly stated responsibilities. They have become obligatory and short-term". In the following, the specific responsibilities of both commissioners and providers are outlined.

Commissioners in local authorities are responsible for the allocation and monitoring of contracts with service providers (Vincent-Jones 2006: 170–171; Seymour 2010). Hence, the commissioner establishes and shapes social care markets, "exercised through their commissioning powers", as described by Knapp *et al.* (2001: 285). The way such commissioning power is used carries long-term implications for both providers and clients: commissioners choose between competing providers on behalf of clients to whom services are ultimately delivered, and who, in market terms, are "the ultimate consumers" (Vincent-Jones 2006: 181, 204). Commissioners are required to assess the client group's needs and to ensure that there are an appropriate number and a range of services available from care providers (Vincent-Jones 2006: 168; Seymour 2010).

Commissioners manage contracts and decide with whom, and on what terms, to contract (Vincent-Jones 2006: 185, 187); although clients are increasingly involved in the development of contracts – this is referred to as "client-based commissioning" (Sheaff *et al.* 2014). Once allocated, the contract needs to be monitored in terms of how service providers fulfil their contractual obligations (Juhila and Günther 2013). In short, commissioners are expected to maximise two goals: minimise cost and maximise the quantity and quality of services purchased (Lane 1999: 187). To a certain extent, commissioners can exercise discretion regarding how to perform their designated commissioning function within local authorities. However, as Vincent-Jones (2006: 188) notes, commissioners' discretion is exercised within the limits of central standards and guidelines favouring certain competitive processes and restricted options.

Providers are responsible for delivering the services as defined in the contract. Knapp *et al.* (2001: 289) note that the externalisation of services from local authorities has shifted "responsibility for achieving externally set standards of care onto the new owners" – the providers. This includes being accountable for the price and quality of their services by reporting and displaying everyday work according to the needs of the purchaser (Meagher and Healy 2003; Saario and Raitakari 2010; Juhila and Günther 2013). In other words, providers are expected to anticipate and offer "value for money" (Dyb and Loison 2007: 134). Within the process of service delivery, the contracts explicate service providers' obligations to produce specified services for a certain group and amount of citizens (Lane 1999). Providers also need to engage in competitive tenders to obtain the necessary funding for their activities (Dyb and Loison 2007: 135). This means that the responsibilities of the service providers vary between particular phases of the commissioning process: in the tender, they have to promise to fulfil the requirements included in the call; while in service delivery, where they are contracted as providers, they must redeem those promises.

Contractual implication and re-responsibilisation of providers

We use the concept of "contractual implication" to point out the formative and consequential nature of commissioning for service providers. One of its consequences can be described by the concept of re-responsibilisation of providers. Both contractual implication and re-responsibilisation originate from governmentality literature, where they are recognised as a part of Rose's (1999) notion on advanced liberalism. We also draw on a currently popular welfare discourse of recovery, which is discussed in more detail in Chapter 3. Together these three concepts provide a frame to analyse providers' responsibilities in commissioning from the point of view of predefined time periods and sanctions that are laid out in contracts.

The concept of contractual implication was originally described by Donzelot (1991). Burchell (1996) uses the concept to refer to a process that brings civil society (the field where NGOs originated and are still often situated) within the sphere of governing. The process takes place by offering individuals and collectivities active involvement in action to resolve the kind of issues hitherto held to be the responsibility of authorized governmental agencies. However, the price for this involvement is that they must assume active responsibility for these activities, both for carrying them out and, of course, for their outcomes, and in so doing they are required to conduct themselves in accordance with the appropriate model of action. This might be described as a new form of "responsibilization" corresponding to the new forms in which the governed are encouraged, freely and rationally, to conduct themselves.

(Burchell 1996: 29)

In the above quote, contracts are viewed as forms of governing technologies affecting the duties, rights and conduct of those involved (Rose 1999; Chapter 2 of this volume). Contractual implication signifies expectations on providers in order to win a contract. It links to "new contractualism", which aims to direct social policy at fostering responsible behaviour (Jayasuriya 2001) and thus points to Miller and Rose's (2008) idea of "governing from the distance", where providers are steered by the contracts "with an expectation that they produce information that makes this steering possible" (Chapter 2; see also Osborne and Gaebler 1993). Lane (1999: 180) envisaged a "contracting state", where resources are to be managed by means of a series of contracts that clarify objectives and tasks for service delivery. Therefore, the commissioning process places more power with the commissioners, and the providers increasingly have to take on the commissioners' expectations in order to win the contract (Kolthoff *et al.* 2007).

One essential implication of commissioning based on contracts can be described as "re-responsiblization of providers". Usually the concept of re-responsiblization is applied to irresponsible citizens or clients (Chapter 2), but in this chapter re-responsibilisation is less about individuals and more about how service-providing organisations are re-responsibilised through contracts. In line with Nilssen and Kildal (2009: 316), it is presumed that providers' "responsible behaviour" can be acquired through a cocktail of sanctions and incentives: the "bindingness" of the contract (Vincent-Jones 2006: 192). Sanctions function as re-responsiblization techniques when providers are not fulfilling their contractual responsibilities – for example, not meeting targets of clients moving on, which can result in the termination of the contract and decommission. At the same time, Rees (2014: 60) describes "risk dumping" as the process of increased transfer of risks and expectations to service providers through the operationalisation of the contract.

Recovery as welfare discourse relates to expectations towards providers, especially timewise. The logic of contracts seems to build on the idea of "recovery from", where a client returning to a healthier state transfers to less intrusive support. However, missing from the logic of contracts is the idea of "recovery in", which emphasises the acceptance of an ongoing presence of an illness, vulnerability to relapse and appropriate support if it occurs, while the client remains in control of his/her own life (Davidson and Roe 2007). Critics of "recovery from" discourse warn about over-optimistic thinking of speedy recovery and setting inappropriate expectations on individuals (Chapter 3). This theme rises in the interviews analysed in this chapter: instead of long-term or permanent support, commissioning calls for client progression by setting up transient and short-term services. Fixed-term contracts provide support within a predefined time set, after which the clients should move on, preferably to a lighter and cheaper service.

Policy reforms in England and Finland have been underpinned by a rehabilitation model that assumes a shift towards independent living can be achieved through strategic planning and a needs-led approach to service provision (O'Malley and Croucher 2005: 832). There is a clear tension present for service providers, who previously provided long-term forms of accommodation having to adopt notions of transitional residences to prepare people for more independent lives. A literature review on supported housing for people with mental health problems displays the popularity of a transitional model from high-intensity support to more independent living (O'Malley and Croucher 2005: 839). The question remains: how to balance the drive for independent living with some people's needs for permanent, high-level support (O'Malley and Croucher 2005: 841)? Juhila *et al.* (2015: 7) note that "in social rehabilitation work, which relies on the linear discourse of time, preferable time arrows show upwards and indicate positive changes and directions in clients' future lives, while descending or horizontal arrows symbolize failures of stagnations" (see also Fahlgren 2009). The NGOs' responsibilities are to promote these preferable futures by rehabilitating clients so that the predefined time limit can be realised and lighter support can take place. Success in fulfilling this responsibility guarantees continuity for the provider by the extension of contract as an incentive (see also Juhila *et al.* 2015: 23).

Accountability and resistance in key stakeholders' talk

The settings situated at the margins of welfare services consist of four NGOs that provide supported housing and floating support for people with mental health and substance abuse problems. Two of the NGOs are Finnish and two are English. The NGOs are in a similar situation regarding their status as providers: their services are commissioned in a quasi-market environment based on the purchaser–provider model. Hence, as described by Vincent-Jones (2006: 167), each of the NGOs operates in "a contractual purchaser–provider relationship".

Lane (1999: 190–191) predicted nearly 20 years ago that the contracting and reviewing of providers in social care would not be applied smoothly due to its "urgency in need" and its "mixture of quantity and quality that often defies definition", and in particular in regard to balancing the tension between price and quality (Wistow *et al.* 1992; Meagher and Healy 2003; van Slyke 2006). The tension is even more difficult to solve in the services situated at the margins of welfare, because these services are targeted at the most vulnerable citizens, with particularly long-term or persistent problems.

To open up the nature of responsibilities in the occasioned commissioning practices, the analysis focuses on service providers' responsibilities as they are constructed in the talk of three key stakeholders: commissioners who purchase the

services, managers of NGOs that provide the services, and, finally, care coordinators who have a distinct role in mediating between these two parties as they
coordinate the support for their clients. The interview data, collected in 2011–2015,
includes altogether 13 interviews of NGO managers, commissioners and care coordinators. There are equal numbers of interviews with managers and commissioners
from Finland and England, while all the interviews with care coordinators are from
England, as there exists no equivalent care coordinator designation in Finland. Furthermore, some commissioning documents are examined to get background
information, such as calls for tenders by purchasers and offers made by providers.

The ways that stakeholders identify providers' responsibilities in interview situations are approached by two analytic concepts: accountability and resistance. In
line with Matarese and Caswell (2014), accountability is approached from the discourse perspective, employing a bottom-up view on accountability as achievements
of everyday talk (Brodkin 2008). As such, the approach differs from the notion of
accountability as a top-down policy concept, focusing instead on those occasions
where people provide reasons for their behaviour in text, talk and interaction
(Chapter 4). Accountability means that people are held responsible – account-able
– for their actions (Garfinkel 1967: 1) and is hence tied to the social and moral
order (Matarese and Caswell 2014: 47; Chapter 4 of this volume). Accountability
becomes visible especially when people explain "the gap between action and
expectation" (Scott and Lyman 1968: 46). Explaining the gap signals that one has
not fulfilled the expected contractual responsibilities (as outlined in contracts) or
has failed to meet them. "Failures" can be explained by justifying, excusing or
blaming (Chapter 4, citing Scott and Lyman 1968). Commissioning carries certain
kinds of moral expectations on different stakeholders' characteristics and responsibilities. For example, NGO managers are expected to be productive (e.g. keeping
"the care promise" made in tender), and failing to meet these expectations requires
displays of accountability.

Resistance is approached as stakeholders' opposition to governmental and institutional policies guiding commissioning (Juhila *et al.* 2014: 124–126). For instance,
the aims of progress in the contract can be criticised as unrealistic, and thus
demands cast for service-providing workers and clients are impossible to fulfil
(Chapter 4). Resistance is also viewed as providers displaying misalignment to
certain institutional purposes of commissioning, such as efficient turnover of
clients, while they can share some other purposes of commissioning, such as the
quality of support.

Service providers' responsibilities in commissioning

Expectations laid out by the commissioning system

This section illustrates the responsibilities that commissioners and providers
manage through commissioning arrangements. We will describe commissioners'
expectations on client turnover, and the predefined time limits for service provision and creating movement through the service system.

Extract 1

COMMISSIONER: Along with the Supporting People grant, we had to issue each one of the homes with contracts, and that was back in 2003. But since then, obviously we've carried out a series of reviews in these services and some of the ones who weren't really up to our expectations, our standards, or we didn't think were meeting a need and demand, then we decommissioned a number of those, and we recommissioned new services as well, where we maybe noticed gaps that weren't being filled and so, some of them are inherited services and some of them are ones where we've actually gone out to, we've identified the need ourselves and we've gone out to, you know, competitive environment what we wanted and ...

(Interview in England 2011)

Here the commissioner in an English local authority describes the development of commissioning. The Supporting People programme (Cameron *et al.* 2007; Buckingham 2009) sets out the responsibility for housing support for vulnerable groups, including those with mental health problems, as a means of enabling independent living. Many of the same providers continued to be funded with contracts "rolled over" rather than put out to tender. As the commissioner notes, however, the change from grants to contracts sets out more clearly the providers' expectations (Rees *et al.* 2014: 18). As the system developed, though, the commissioner began to review whether the "inherited" range of provision was appropriate for the client population's needs. An active orientation to developing the social care market is described: a concern with "*standards*", "*meeting a need and demand*", "*noticed gaps*", which resulted in decommissioning and recommissioning some services. The commissioner embraces the advantages of "*identifying the need ourselves*" and going out into the "*competitive environment (for) what we wanted*". There are all the elements of what Rees (2014: 48) calls the "commissioning cycle".

Once the contract has been enacted, the commissioner has a number of means for monitoring the service provided, such as annual reviews:

Extract 2

COMMISSIONER: Well, what we do is we do an annual review, of these services, and when we do that review, we'll look at the support plans and make sure that they, like, contain smart objectives, that there, contains things that we want to see in there, such as the need for the person to move on, and they're looking at the outcomes that we've said that we want them to achieve, such as help supporting people into work, like, training, education, better managing their physical health and things like; that so we check the support plans to ensure they're doing those things.

(Interview in England 2011)

In the annual review, the commissioner has the right and responsibility to examine the clients' support plans and to look for evidence that objectives for encouraging moves to greater independence are included. Here, the commissioner expects to find documented evidence that the clients are directed to move on and that the service provider is "*looking at the outcomes*". This is to be found not merely in the support for housing, but also in action taken to promote the clients' engagement with training and education as well as with self-management (see Chapter 5).

Extract 3

COMMISSIONER: We keep an idea on the turnover. You know I said that providers fill out each week, to say who's on their waiting list and things like that? They also fill out a form to say who they've got ready to move on from the service and then we'll prompt them and, to say: are they registered with choice-based lettings to be able to bid for their own accommodation, are they looking at private, are they registered with the other housing associations? And when we do our, like annual review of the service, we'll ask the question about who's looking in the accommodation, how long have you been there, are you working with a care coordinator, to constantly ask if the person's ready to move on.

(Interview in England 2011)

In response to the interviewer's question about turnover, that is, clients moving on and therefore creating vacancies for others, the commissioner describes a system of weekly monitoring of vacancies and waiting lists. Again the active encouragement from the commissioner is apparent through his checking that appropriate steps are being followed by the service provider: are clients "*ready to move on*", in other words, are they registered with potential housing providers? There is further questioning of whether the practitioners are adequately working together, since once the client is considered "ready to move" the onus moves to the care coordinator to manage the next move. The commissioner places responsibility on the service providers to instigate the next move, and sees them as accountable for assessing and recording the clients' readiness to move on to more independent housing, although formally it is the care coordinator who oversees the care plan and who therefore manages any moving on. Below, the commissioner reports other activity to manage the system and keep the clients moving.

Extract 4

COMMISSIONER: And also on the number of people they've had referred to the service, so we can see where the demands are. On the number of people who are waiting to move on from services. So that we can identify if there's any bottlenecks, why people aren't moving on if somebody's been there a while; we'll try and step in and say "is there anything we can do to help them move on"?

(Interview in England 2012)

The commissioner aims to manage the system as a whole by contracting for services where there are heavy demands. However, in order to keep the supply and demand for appropriate places, they have to monitor "*bottlenecks*". In the tender, providers have to make certain promises to promote the client's progress or "recovery". Hence, the key responsibility that falls on providers is to move their clients to other services offering lighter support within a predetermined time period stated in the contract. Being responsible for the movement of clients, they are expected to achieve a certain turnover rate, and yet as mentioned above, the service providers might have to wait for the care coordinator to achieve the next move. The latter can be seen as an example of risk dumping (Rees 2014: 60).

Extract 5

COMMISSIONER: This [care promise system] is how we aim to reach effectiveness, because what we've had before in these mental health services was that our commissioners have to run around all the time and, in a way, kick clients forward, and, in a way, here we kind of move that responsibility to service providers so that it will be in their own interest to move clients forward. So, if they do it really well, they will have a really long contract and it will be, in a way, in their own interest. And then again, if they don't do it, but they store them, putting it ugly, store the clients, they won't be up to this so this will, in a way, make things easier for the municipality.

(Interview in Finland 2013)

This extract from Finland displays the "care promise" that providers need to include in their tendering bid. The care promise signifies that the provider promises to move on a certain percentage of their clients to a lighter form of support within a predetermined time period. Here, "the recovery" is operationalised in a way that, during a one-year period, the client can move to a lighter support and stay there for at least three months. Within this particular call for tender, the minimum promise allowed for provider candidates was 20 per cent of clients, resulting in providers' bids ranging from 30 to 70 per cent. Breaking the care promise signifies sanctions directed at providers: if providers fail to deliver the care promise in two consecutive years, they are sanctioned by decommission. Redeeming the promise is rewarded by bonuses. The bonus for the two providers who reach the highest percentages is a continued contract, so after the first contract (four years plus a two-year option), they will get another four years and two-year option, without taking part in a competitive tender.

Overall, this section has shown the commissioners' active involvement in establishing tendering processes and awarding contracts, but it has also shown the ongoing activity to monitor and encourage, sometimes on a weekly basis, the operation of the social care market. As Rees *et al.* (2014: 14) note, "feedback mechanisms and channels for dialogue occur through a wider variety of ways that would not necessarily be regarded as part of commissioning". The central concern is "moving on", both in terms of the individual client's progress to greater independence, and also in ensuring that new clients can access the system and that the service providers' units are working at maximum capacity. Recovery is used to drive all of these objectives.

Challenging the time limits within commissioning by subtle resistance

This second stage of our analysis will provide a detailed examination of the discursive construction of providers' responsibilities. We look at the reactions of care coordinators and service providers to the time limits of commissioning outlined in the previous subsection, drawing on the concepts of resistance, accountability, justification and responsibilities. In the extracts below, interviewees are accounting for not achieving certain aims of commissioning, such as the desired turnover or progress of clients. There is a gap between the provider's own action (not progressing the clients to a lighter support) and the commissioners' expectation (clients should be forwarded to a less-supported service within a defined time limit) (Scott and Lyman 1968, 46, ref. Chapter 4; Matarese and Caswell 2014). In our data we see patterns of resistance by interviewees in implicit ways, using the following contrasts: ideal vs. realistic; high level vs. low level; short term vs. long term; recovery from vs. recovery in; and young people vs. others. All these contrasts can be understood as linked to accountability.

Prior to the extract below, the care coordinator talks about cuts in social services and how the contracting system is outcome based, which puts pressure on providers to move clients to less intensive, cheaper services within two years.

Extract 6

CARE COORDINATOR: We have quite a high proportion of relatively young individuals with particularly severe and chronic mental health problems, where to remain stable they need, in the community, to have a quality life, they require quite a high level of support. Now, that high level of support can be found in Supporting People accommodation, but only for two years. Then, after that, it's a low level of support. Now, for some of these people they are at their optimum, and any less is failure, which has been proven with several of our clients, but then you can't keep them there forever. So it's either there or residential care. There seems to be a bit of a gap in what can be provided. So increasingly we're now having – I mean, I work with a guy who's now 33 year old and in a residential nursing home, and he wants all the things out of life that a 33 year old would want, but you're not going to get that in a residential home, are you, unfortunately. So we're having to make some kind of quite unpleasant life choices for people.

INTERVIEWER: And would he function in somewhere like [name of the NGO]?

CARE COORDINATOR: Not [name of the NGO] necessarily, but he would function in a higher level 24-hour. But realistically, both I know, his family knows, and he knows, more importantly, that actually he wouldn't be able to cope in two years' time, or even four or five years' time, with that kind of low

level of support. So I guess we've just cut out the middle man and gone to residential care, because that was, he came from hospital, but we were then – I would ideally, because of his age, be looking at a less intense environment for that. But we know that he's not going to manage to do that, and then in two years' time, take a step down again. He's always, realistically we all know that he's always going to require quite a high level of support.
INTERVIEWER: OK.

(Interview in England 2013)

In this extract the care coordinator voices a subtle resistance towards the commissioning system. The resistance is directed towards the two-year limit and the required movement for clients. The care coordinator initially points out that a substantial proportion of the clients are young people with severe and chronic problems. This poses a problem, as they need a high level of support, but amongst the services contracted by the municipality, high-level support is available only for two years, which is not enough for these clients. He talks of this restriction in an accepting manner as he says "*… but then you can't keep them there forever*", "there" presumably being the high-level care. He points out a problem inherent in this: "*There seems to be a bit of a gap in what can be provided*". While stating the problem, the care coordinator does not direct blame explicitly towards anyone in particular, nor does he state who is responsible for the problem. Instead he distances the problem by balancing between what "*we*" can do and what is available in the system. The gap between what can be provided on the one hand, and what is needed on the other, is accounted for by twice using the words "*we are … having to*". This constraint and the shared responsibility ("we" rather than "I") work to mitigate any possible blame for not being able to close this gap. The care coordinator addresses the contrast between high and low levels of support. High-level support is depicted as positive, using expressions such as "*remain stable*", "*quality of life*" and "*at their optimum*". High-level support is possible amongst contracted services but limited to a two-year maximum. In the policy documents, low-level support is defined as the ideal form of support. However, in the extract above, the care coordinator recognises the particular client group of younger people with chronic and severe problems as problematic in terms of low-level support: "*any less is failure*".

The care coordinator illustrates the problematics with an example of a 33-year-old man. In this example, moving from a high to a low level of support is not deemed possible: "*But realistically, both I know, his family knows, and he knows, more importantly, that actually he wouldn't be able to cope in two years' time, or even four or five years' time, with that kind of low level of support*". The ideal view of progression of clients from high- to low-level support within a timeframe of two years as defined in the policy documents is not possible. Instead, a different option is used: a long-term "*residential nursing home*", which is seen as "*unfortunate*" and "*unpleasant*" but which is available even though the client is unable to make the "recovery from". In other words, the "unfortunate and unpleasant" choice of long-term residential care for this particular client can be seen as a perverse effect of the contractual system and a consequence of the gap between the ideal of "recovery from" and progression as defined in policy documents on the one hand, and the reality of the client group on the other. The distinction between high-level and low-level support is one contrast at play here. Another contrast, however, is also present in the talk, namely the distinction between short-term and long-term care. For this client, long-term care is not a preferred option. In order for him to get long-term care on more than a low level of support, the care coordinator has found it necessary to move him to residential care.

Another contrast that surfaces in the data is the distinction between realistic and ideal. The care coordinator's justification uses the above example of the 33-year-old client "*... in a residential nursing home, and he wants all the things out of life that a 33-year old would want, but you're not going to get that in a residential home, are you, unfortunately*". He is stating that the ideal is to have "*the things out of life that a 33-year old would want*", but he dismisses this as unrealistic. The ideal vs. reality distinction is age-related, as the client group consists of a high proportion of young people with severe and chronic problems. While ideally the support provided would aim at enabling clients to have a similar lifestyle to belong to people of a similar age, realistically this is limited by the available support. The option of residential care as a long-term solution also implies dilemmas, as the "young clients" will be offered support within a social work framework mainly aimed at older people. The dilemma of age also relates to the general expectation that young people ideally are expected to recover from their present life situation. When such an ideal development does not occur, it undermines the support system, as well as the client's progress. The dilemma for the care coordinator is that he might know what the client needs but be unable to provide it. The ideal of movement, progression and recovery as addressed in policy (and thus inherent in the commissioning system) is not a reality of this client group. This gap poses dilemmas for the individual client, but also prompts the care coordinator to provide accounts in the shape of justifications and excuses.

A few minutes later in the interview, the care coordinator continues to examine dilemmas inherent in supported housing within the commissioning arrangement.

Extract 7

INTERVIEWER: And when you've got someone in a more supported housing and the two years are coming up, what's the pressure that's being put on you?

CARE COORDINATOR: Quite a lot, actually. Because they have the link person from social services who deals with Supporting People, who's talking about funding, and that's their job to kind of ensure that they're getting value for money and moving people on to a less expensive environment. So they are, if you were doing this research with a lot of the, say [name of an NGO] and [name of an NGO], they could tell you themselves that they are getting constant pressure, weekly, they have to give a weekly report about moving on, and that then filters back to me. I get a lot of pressure about what am I doing to find them somewhere, and as I said, we have a few clients who there is nowhere else for them, that's as good as it's going to be.

INTERVIEWER: And if that comes about – I mean, I think, I know that sometimes people get a slight extension, but it's only going to be a couple of months, from what I gather.

CARE COORDINATOR: Yeah, I mean you can have – there's a guy who I work with who's ...

[Talking about who the particular client is]

CARE COORDINATOR: Now he's moving on shortly, but he's had an extension of a year. But the thing is, they know that they're on borrowed time, that's the thing as well. And now, he's now, relapse signatures are coming through because of the stress of the moving. And he will continue – it'll be constant unsettlement. He always knows that he's going, the expectation is moving on. He can't put down roots.

(Interview in England 2013)

In this extract the care coordinator points out how different actors have different responsibilities within the commissioning system. The "*link person from social services*" (probably the commissioner) is responsible for getting "*value for money*", which is defined here as ensuring that clients are moved on to less expensive supported housing. The NGOs delivering supported housing, on the other hand, have different responsibilities. One of these is "*to give a weekly report*" – that is, to document the clients' progress. The care coordinator has yet another responsibility, namely to "*find them somewhere*". This latter responsibility relates to finding the best possible supported housing for the individual client within the restrictions imposed by the system. As such, the care coordinator talks of his role as only partly accountable, because the system restricts his actions. He accounts for his actions by describing himself as being under "*a lot of pressure*". He uses justification as an accountability strategy when talking about the dilemma between, on the one hand, knowing the client and his/her needs and, on the other hand, knowing that supported housing is only temporary and that the client will have to be moved on; as he says: "*the expectation is moving on*". While he will have the possibility to postpone this move in particular situations where this is deemed beneficial to the client, this is only temporary. The example of a particular male client challenges the optimistic idea of speedy recovery within limited time frames inherent in the commissioning system of supported housing. Rather than supporting the client in a recovery process, the care coordinator talks of how "*relapse signatures are coming through because of the stress of the moving*". He is able to question the general tenets of the recovery-based commissioning system by noting exigencies faced by particular clients.

The next extract is from the Finnish NGO, which has undergone a rapid change from being a voluntary and grant-based organisation to being a service provider within the new commissioning system. It was established as a local, community-based response to a rapid reduction in hospital beds in the area, which had resulted in a lack of supported housing for those discharged. The NGO was set up to provide such housing, along with day activities and work-related rehabilitation. The overall aims were to provide "homes for life", to promote the users' human rights and to create a sense of community. Funding was provided by three parties: the Finnish Slot Machine Association; the Common Responsibility Campaign, an annual fundraising scheme organised by the Finnish Lutheran Church; and the city council. The major change that brought the NGO into the sphere of commissioning was the introduction of the Public Procurement Act, along with the simultaneous establishment of the local purchaser–provider model; both require the NGO to enter into the established social care market or to withdraw from running supported housing completely. Here the NGO manager talks about the clients' progression as central to the current commissioning system. She provides an example of a "care promise" to describe clients' turnover expectations.

Extract 8

INTERVIEWER: A couple of years ago it was quite a different tender, compared to this new one, I mean back in 2013 there was the care promise, isn't that right?

MANAGER: Yeah, back then we had to put the exact percentage, we had to put the number of people who would move to a lighter [support] during a calendar year and we put the promise of 30 per cent then – we thought that three out of ten people could be thought to be able to move on. Well we didn't even get close to that. And you know, [another NGO in the area] had put 55 per cent and it went really wrong for them; it just doesn't work in practice, because what happened with them [the other provider] was that they were persuaded to take this one client who is a really difficult case – that "please just take this person to your supported housing, to test and try it out", so that you could see whether he can cope with your support. This client was then included in the 55 per cent, of course, and now that they've failed to move [this client] to a lighter support so they are now threatened, they now have to pay the penalty. In the end, you cannot decide for yourself who is taken in the service, but it is the [the local commissioning agency] who decide, and then you cannot reach your goal, the goal you yourself have established and counted to be probable. And all the time these clients are getting more and more difficult.

(Interview in Finland 2015)

This extract displays criticism towards the "care promise" in the Finnish tender, which was described by the Finnish commissioner in Extract 5. In this extract we see a similar contrast to the one in the previous data from the English case between the ideal of "*being able to move on*" and the reality that "*clients are getting more and more difficult*". The NGO manager questions the required movement within the predetermined time frame. She points to a particular example of a service provider currently in a threatened situation, which has to pay a penalty for failing to achieve the target of moving clients on. The NGO manager talks of the complex responsibility in this situation. While the service providers are responsible for setting targets, which may or may not be realistic, it is not the service providers themselves who are solely responsible for which clients they have to work with. In this particular case the service provider "*was persuaded to take this one ... really difficult case*", which contributes to the ambitions target being out of reach. The responsibility of which clients are offered which services lies with the local commissioning agency, as there are no nominated care coordinators to decide which provider to approach.

The resistance in this extract is more overt than in the previous sections, deploying upgraded terms: "*it went really wrong*", "*it doesn't work*" and "*they failed*". The key message from the NGO manager is that the targets that were set were unrealistic and the price for not meeting targets harsh. The resistance is also related to the client group. As in the previous extract, there seems to be a contrast between the ideal and the real client group. This ideal client is in line with a neoliberal perspective, with the idea of "recovery from" and development as a linear progression. The real client group, on the other hand, is much more complex and difficult, causing problems for progression. Consequently such clients struggle to meet targets, and both clients and service providers pay the price for this mismatch. The knowledge that the "ideal client" does not match the real clients seems to be shared knowledge amongst both service providers and commissioners, who persuade service providers to take difficult clients. The failure to move clients forward to the extent defined in the care promise does not seem to be a big surprise. In the example above, the "persuasion" of the service provider indicates that this particular client is expected to pose a challenge to them. Nonetheless, the responsibility for failure falls on the service provider, as they are unable to meet the targets they themselves have set (and possibly on the client, but this is not addressed in the extract). In the extract there is a tension in regard to the appropriateness of the placement for the individual client and the pressure to accept the placement suggested by the local commissioning agency. The NGO manager reports the words (Holt and Clift 2007) of the commissioner by saying "*please just take this person to your supported housing, to test and try it out*". Using the words "*please*", "*just*" and "*test and try*" works to mitigate the possible problems this situation might raise. As such, the NGO presents the local commissioning agency as having almost tricked the service provider into taking the client, and then when (as possibly expected) they fail to move the client forward to a lighter support, the consequences are not mitigated.

The NGO manager is implying that providers are placed in a difficult situation within the tendering process. The targets are set within a competitive situation of winning the tender. Once these targets are set, they form a care promise that the service providers must live up to. If this is not achieved, sanctions are being used, such as threats and penalties embedded in the contract. The NGO manager voices resistance towards the pattern of sanctions. She points out two problems: the local commissioning agency being in charge of deciding which clients are offered which services, and the client group becoming increasingly difficult. However, while voicing resistance, she also puts forward how it is a challenge in the tendering process to make ambitious but not completely unrealistic targets – a challenge her own NGO managed with greater success than the other service provider in her example. Her NGO had set an ambitious target of moving three out of ten clients forward, but "*didn't even get close to that*". This is, however, less of a failure than the situation facing the other service provider, which set an even more ambitious target of "*55 per cent and it went really wrong for them*". The ability of service providers to balance the ambitious with the realistic and possible is essential, since when they set the goals for themselves, they need to anticipate the competition in order to go through the tendering process successfully.

Conclusion and discussion

This chapter has focused on key professional stakeholders within the commissioning process, including commissioners, service provider managers and care coordinators. Through the analysis of their interviews, we have illustrated the complex construction of service providers' responsibilities within local practices of commissioning services for the marginalised client groups.

The first part of the analysis focused on the expectations laid out by the commissioning system. There we saw how the provision of supported housing is directed by a commissioning cycle: the municipality assesses the client population's needs, develops a commissioning strategy which envisages a range of service provision, procures such services through tendering and contracting and, finally, monitors and reviews the balance between the supply of places and demand of clients. (Rees *et al.* 2014: 15). While it is constructed as a social care market, the commissioners do not merely leave the market to work by themselves on the basis that supply and demand will produce some form of equilibrium. Through the terms of the contract, a range of sanctions and encouragements are established regarding how a service is to be provided as well as the expectations of client outcomes. In particular, the commissioning system is based on a notion of client progress and movement that draws on "recovery". Furthermore, the commissioners continually check that all parties remain on course to keep clients moving through the system, both in terms of stated goals and achieved performances. In these ways, the responsibilities for success and failure are established and allocated to clients and service providers.

The second part of the analysis concentrated on how key professional stakeholders justify, account for and resist the commissioning system. A range of criticisms and subtle forms of resistance are voiced by service providers and care coordinators towards the commissioning system. Although none overtly challenge the policy ambitions for clients to progress from higher to lower levels of support and cheaper services, a strong contrast is made between ideal progress through the system and the reality for many clients. Two contrasts are drawn on, in particular between the expectations of the commissioning system and everyday dilemmas of service providers and care coordinators: high-level versus low-level support, and short-term versus long-term support. The responsibility of providers regarding making promises on clients moving on within a predefined time limit was constructed as problematic. For some clients, such time frames were considered unrealistic. Furthermore, the range of provider services is not at an appropriate level of support to suit some clients. Other contrasts pertaining to clients include "recovery from" versus "recovery in", and young people versus others. All these contrasts can be understood as being linked to attempts to manage accountability in complex ways, as service providers and care coordinators resist notions that policies can be implemented in straightforward ways associated with presuppositions of a smooth "recovery journey" (Leamy *et al.* 2011) for clients who pose risks and challenges.

The detailed analysis of interview talk of professional stakeholders reveals some nuances and contingencies within the commissioning system that tend to remain unnoticed at the systemic level (Maynard-Moody and Musheno 2003; Brodkin 2008). These include the "perverse effects" of contractual procedures, where policies produce unintended consequences for everyday practices, often resulting in resistance performed by front-line workers (Thomas and Davies 2005; Saario 2012). One unintended consequence within commissioning concerns NGOs having to compromise their mission to enter the contracting process. The assumption that clients will progress from higher to lower levels of support is especially problematic, making it increasingly difficult for providers to respond to the needs of those who require long-term accommodation with high levels of support (see also O'Malley and Croucher 2005: 831). Similar contradictions between efficiency and clients' needs or preferences are recognised in market-driven services (e.g. Vincent-Jones 2006: 199; Harlock 2014; Jantz *et al.* 2015). "The era of austerity" causes evident pressure to procure the services that primarily offer value for money (Rees *et al.* 2014). In the interviews, NGO managers criticise commissioning for being primarily focused on procurement and prices, while some parts of the commissioning cycle, such as the assessment of local population needs in collaboration with providers, seem to be missing (see also Rees 2014: 48–50, 60).

As pointed out above, contractual procedures are essential in commissioning. The contract defines and allocates responsibilities for providers by outlining the contents, prices and time frames for services. Accordingly, the contract is recognised as a technology that directs the activities of providers and therefore carries major contractual implications (Burchell 1996; Sending and Neumann 2006; Saario 2014). From this perspective, the contract directs providers by what Miller and Rose (2008) term as "governing at a distance": while clearly being directed by commissioning, providers still remain spatially and organisationally distinct from the commissioning agency. Even though the contract specifies a wide range of reviews and reporting systems, to ensure that the provider is performing as agreed, everyday practices of support work are independently conducted by the service provider staff. In this way, the contract features providers as "quasi-autonomous entities", having both autonomising and responsibilising effects (Rose *et al.* 2006: 91). The interviewees seem to address commissioning primarily in terms of regulation and new managerial responsibilities, even though the original aim of quasi-markets was to move social care towards deregulation (Vincent-Jones 2006: 198). Governing providers at a distance thus signifies less discretion, and more assigning of responsibilities and accounting for their performance and outcomes (Rose *et al.* 2006).

References

Alcock, P. (2010) "Building the Big Society: a new policy environment for the third sector in England", *Voluntary Sector Review*, 1(3): 379–389.

Bayard, J., Calianno, C. and Mee, C. (1997) "Care coordinator: blending roles to improve patient outcomes", *Nursing Management*, 28(8): 49–52.

Bode, I., Gardin, L. and Nyssens, M. (2011) "Quasi-marketisation in domiciliary care: varied patterns, similar problems?", *International Journal of Sociology and Social Policy*, 31(3/4): 222–235.

Bovaird, T., Dickinson, H. and Allen, K. (2012) *Commissioning across Government: Review of evidence*. Project Report. Birmingham: University of Birmingham.

Brodkin, E. (2008) "Accountability in street-level organizations", *International Journal of Public Administration*, 31(3): 317–336.

Buckingham, H. (2009) "Competition and contracts in the voluntary sector: exploring the implications for homelessness service providers in Southampton", *Policy and Politics*, 37(2): 235–254.

Burchell, G. (1996) "Liberal government and techniques of the self", in A. Barry, T. Osborne and N. Rose (eds), *Foucault and Political Reason: Liberalism, neo-liberalism and rationalities of government* (pp. 19–36), Chicago: University of Chicago Press.

Cameron, A., MacDonald, G., Turner, W. and Lloyd, L. (2007) "The challenges of joint working: lessons from the Supporting People Health Pilot evaluation", *International Journal of Integrated Care*, 7(18), 1–10.

Carmel, E. and Harlock, J. (2008) "Instituting the 'third sector' as a governable terrain: partnership, procurement and performance in the UK", *Policy & Politics*, 36(2): 155–171.

Cunningham, I. and James, P. (2009) "The outsourcing of social care in Britain: what does it mean for voluntary sector workers?", *Work Employment & Society*, 23(2): 363–375.

Davidson, L. and Roe, D. (2007) "Recovery from versus recovery in serious mental illness: one strategy for lessening confusion plaguing recovery", *Journal of Mental Health*, 16(4): 459–470.

Donzelot, J. (1991) *Face à L'exclusion,* Paris: Ed. Esprit.

Dufva, V. (2005) "Sosiaali- ja terveysjärjestöperheet kuvassa" [Social and health care NGOs in the family portrait], in J. Niemelä and V. Dufva (eds) *Hyvinvoinnin arjen asiantuntijat: Sosiaali- ja terveysjärjestöt uudella vuosituhannella* [Experts of everyday welfare: social and health care NGOs in the new millennium] (pp. 11–27), Jyväskylä, Finland: PS-kustannus.

Dyb, E. and Loison, M. (2007) "Impact of service procurement and competition on quality and standards in homeless service provision", *European Journal of Homelessness*, 1(1): 119–140.

Fahlgren, S. (2009) "Discourse analysis of childcare drama: or the interfaces between paradoxical discourses of time in the context of social work", *Time & Society*, 18(2/3): 208–230.

Garfinkel, H. (1967) *Studies in Ethnomethodology*, Cambridge: Polity Press.

Harlock, J. (2014) "From outcomes-based commissioning to social value? Implications for performance managing the third sector", Working Paper 123, University of Birmingham: Third Sector Research Centre.

Holt, E. and Clift, R. (eds) (2007) *Reporting Talk: Reported speech in interaction*. Cambridge: Cambridge University Press.

Jantz, B., Klenk, T., Larsen, F. and Wiggan, J. (2015) "Marketization and varieties of accountability relationships in employment services: comparing Denmark, Germany, and Great Britain", *Administration & Society*, DOI: 10.1177/0095399715581622.

Jayasuriya, K. (2001) "Autonomy, liberalism and the new contractualism", *Law in Context*, 18(2): 57–78.

Jordan, L. and van Tuijl, P. (2006) *NGO Accountability: Politics, principles and innovations*, London: Earthscan.

Juhila, K., Caswell, D. and Raitakari, S. (2014) "Resistance", in C. Hall, K. Juhila, M. Matarese and C. van Nijnatten (eds) *Analysing Social Work Communication: Discourse in practice* (pp. 117–135), London: Routledge.

Juhila, K. and Günther, K. (2013) "Kunnan, järjestöjen ja asiakkaiden oikeudet ja velvollisuudet tilaaja-tuottajamallissa: tutkimus asumispalvelujen tarjouspyyntöasiakirjoista" [Rights and responsibilities of municipalities, non-governmental organizations and service users in the purchaser–provider model], *Janus*, 21(3): 298–313.

Juhila, K., Günther, K. and Raitakari, S. (2015) "Negotiating mental health rehabilitation plans: joint future talk and clashing time talk in professional client interaction", *Time & Society*, 24(1): 5–26.

Knapp, M., Hardy, B. and Forder, J. (2001) "Commissioning for quality: ten years of social care markets in England", *Journal of Social Policy*, 30(2): 283–306.

Kolthoff, E., Huberts, L. and van den Heuvel, H. (2007) "The ethics of New Public Management: is integrity at stake?", *Public Administration Quarterly*, Winter: 399–439.

Koskiaho, B. (2008) *Hyvinvointipalvelujen tavaratalossa* [In the department store of welfare services], Tampere: Vastapaino.

Koskiaho, B. (2014) *Kumppanuuden sosiaalipolitiikkaa etsimässä* [Searching for social policy of companionship], Helsinki: Setlementtiliitto.

Lane, J.-E. (1999) "Contractualism in the public sector", *Public Management: An International Journal of Research and Theory*, 1(2): 179–194.

Leamy, M., Bird, V., Le Boutillier, C., Williams, C. and Slade, M. (2011) "Conceptual framework for personal recovery in mental health: systematic review and narrative synthesis", *British Journal of Psychiatry*, 199(6): 445–452.

Lundström, T. and Svedberg, L. (2003) "The voluntary sector in a social democratic welfare state: the case of Sweden", *Journal of Social Policy*, 32(2): 217–238.

Matarese, M. and Caswell, D. (2014) "Accountability", in C. Hall, K. Juhila, M. Matarese and C. Van Nijnatten (eds) *Analysing Social Work Communication: Discourse in practice* (pp. 44–60), London: Routledge.

Maynard-Moody, S. and Musheno, M. (2003) *Cops, Teachers, Counselors: Stories from the front lines of public service*, Ann Arbor: University of Michigan Press.

Meagher, G. and Healy, K. (2003) "Caring, controlling, contracting and counting: governments and non-profits in community services", *Australian Journal of Public Administration*, 62(3): 40–51.

Miller, P. and Rose, N. (2008) *Governing the Present: Administering economic, social and personal life*, Cambridge: Polity Press.

Nilssen, E. and Kildal, N. (2009) "New contractualism in social policy and the Norwegian fight against poverty and social exclusion", *Ethics & Social Welfare*, 3(3): 303–321.

O'Malley, L. and Croucher, K. (2005) "Supported housing services for people with mental health problems: a scoping study", *Housing Studies*, 20(5): 831–845.

Onyett, S. (1998) *Case Management in Mental Health*, London: Nelson Thornes.

Osbourne, D. and Gaebler, J. (1993) *Reinventing Government: How the entrepreneurial spirit is transforming the public sector*, New York: Plume.

Rees, J. (2014) "Public sector commissioning and the third sector: old wine in new bottles?", *Public Policy and Administration*, 29(1): 45–63.

Rees, J., Miller, R. and Buckingham, H. (2014) "Public Sector Commissioning of Local Mental Health Services from the Third Sector", Working Paper 122, University of Birmingham: Third Sector Research Centre.

Rose, N. (1999) *Powers of Freedom: Reframing political thought*, Cambridge: Cambridge University Press.

Rose, N., O'Malley, P. and Valverde, M. (2006) "Governmentality", *Annual Review on Law and Social Science*, 2: 83–104.

Rubery, J., Grimshaw, D. and Hebson, G. (2012) "Exploring the limits to local authority social care commissioning: competing pressures, variable practices, and unresponsive providers", *Public Administration*, 91(2): 419–437.

Saario, S. (2012) "Managerial reforms and psychiatric care: a study of resistive practices performed by mental health practitioners", *Sociology of Health and Illness*, 34(6): 896–910.

Saario, S. (2014) *Audit Techniques in Mental Health: Practitioners' responses to electronic health records and service purchasing agreements*, Tampere: Acta Universitatis Tamperensis, 1907.

Saario, S. and Raitakari, S. (2010) "Contractual audit and mental health rehabilitation: a study of formulating effectiveness in a Finnish supported housing unit", *International Journal of Social Welfare*, 19(3): 321–329.

Sánchez Graells, A. (2015) *Public Procurement and the EU Competition Rules*, Second edition, Oxford: Hart Publishing.

Scott, M. and Lyman, S. (1968) "Accounts", *American Sociological Review*, 33(1): 46–62.

Sending, O. and Neumann, I. (2006) "Governance to governmentality: analyzing NGOs, states, and power", *International Studies Quarterly*, 50(3): 651–672.

Seymour, L. (2010) "Commissioning for mental health", *Mental Health Review Journal*, 15(1): 4–9.

Sheaff, R., Charles, N., Mahon, A., Chambers, N., Morando, V., Exworthy, M., Byng, R., Mannion, R. and Llewellyn, S. (2014) "NHS commissioning practice and health system governance: a mixed-methods realistic evaluation", *Health Services and Delivery Research*, 3(10).

Stace, H. and Cumming, J. (2006) "Contracting between government and the voluntary sector: where to from here?' *Policy Quarterly*, 2(4): 13–20.

Thomas, R. and Davies, A. (2005) "Theorizing the micro-politics of resistance: New Public Management and managerial identities in the UK public services", *Organization Studies*, 26(5): 683–706.

Tsui, M.S. and Cheung, F.C.H. (2004) "Gone with the wind: the impacts of managerialism on human services", *British Journal of Social Work*, 34(3): 437–442.

Tynkkynen, L.-K., Keskimäki, I. and Lehto, J. (2013) "Purchaser–provider splits in health care: the case of Finland", *Health Policy*, 111(3): 221–225.

van Slyke, D. (2006) "Agents or stewards: using theory to understand the government–nonprofit social service contracting relationship", *Journal of Public Administration Research and Theory*, 17(2): 157–187.

Vincent-Jones, P. (2006) *The New Public Contracting: Regulation, responsiveness, relationality*, Oxford: Oxford University Press.

Wistow, G., Knapp, M., Hardy, B. and Allen, C. (1992) "From providing to enabling: local authorities and the mixed economy of social care", *Public Administration*, 70(1): 25–45.

11 Conclusions

Suvi Raitakari, Kirsi Juhila and Christopher Hall

Multiple practices of responsibilisation

In this book we have examined talk, text and interactions at the margins of welfare services to widen understandings of how responsibilisation and related welfare discourses might be present, managed and negotiated among clients, welfare workers and managers as part of their everyday practices, and with what consequences. We scrutinised data examples from naturally occurring worker–client encounters, case-planning and team meetings, and interviews with managers, workers and clients, to learn and demonstrate how responsibilities are talked into being as everyday issues that need to be addressed.

We came across demanding, challenging and complicated realities in a variety of institutional settings that provide services for people with complex needs:

- supported housing and floating support services;
- a project offering housing and social skills training for young adults with diagnosed schizophrenia;
- a low-threshold outpatient clinic for people with severe drug abuse problems;
- a prison and probation service.

What is common to these settings is that workers and clients collaborate to tackle the clients' social exclusion, which results from illness, poverty, addiction and/or homelessness. This is done in situations where both the clients and the workers have restricted resources and choices, whose management is consequential and often contested. Hence, these institutions are in many ways perfect settings to study the everyday presence, applicability and challenges of responsibilisation in services targeted at disadvantaged and vulnerable citizens. As we have seen in this book, responsibilisation is especially urgent for those at the margins, whose accountability and responsibility can be questioned when they are faced with demands that draw on advanced liberal thinking.

One of our starting hypotheses was that discourses related to responsibilisation are more critical and consequential for disadvantaged and vulnerable citizens, and for welfare workers encountering them in grass-roots level services, than for better-off, active and healthy citizens. The expectations of responsible citizenship concern everyone, but take on different and stronger resonances at the margins of welfare than in "mainstream society". The second hypothetical starting point was that both the clients and welfare workers are the objects and subjects of (re)-responsibilisation processes that they participate in and resist. Responsibilisation can be seen to affect both parties and to be open to "technologies of self" (e.g. Rose 1990) that are targeted at a "transformation of the self".

Issues related to responsibilisation were addressed in the practices of the settings, and influenced the conduct and self-identities of both the clients and the workers. They could be recognised when the participants negotiated "who will do what" and "who is, or should be, responsible for what" (see Chapter 9). It was also related to discussions on self-determination and becoming the empowered subject of one's life (see Chapter 5). In this sense, it can be said that the ideas of responsibilisation were translated, adjusted, "tamed" and challenged on various occasions in grass-roots level encounters.

Although the issues related to responsibilisation are present in many ways at the margins of welfare services, they are not often available for reflection in any straightforward manner by clients and workers. In ethnomethodological terms they are "seen, but unnoticed" (Garfinkel 1967). To make them more noticed, we examined connections between policy-level discussions on responsibilisation (examined in the governmentality literature) and grass-roots level service practices. Furthermore, we asked how currently influential welfare discourses related to responsibilities are present and oriented to in everyday practices. This connection between policies and practices was developed by following ideas of the turn to researching practices in social and human sciences, and by using mediating analytic concepts that made it possible to examine such talk, text and interaction that may indicate the presence of responsibilisation in grass-roots level welfare services (see Chapter 4).

The main contribution of the book is that it brings more perspectives and nuances to the prevailing policy-level analyses of responsibilisation by demonstrating and problematising the management of responsibilities in everyday welfare services. Each empirical chapter has examined a "big" responsibilisation discourse, which can be identified in particular technologies, techniques, mediating concepts and interactional actions. Responsibilisation is thus understood as multiple, complex and conflicting interactive accomplishments conducted in various institutional settings.

The process of writing the book has made it clear that this kind of ethnomethodologically oriented research has strengths and possibilities but also limitations. Unquestionably, there is a distance between macro-level policies and discourses and micro-level everyday practices. Narrowing this distance requires interpretative imagination and becoming familiar with policies and theories as well as ethnomethodological data analysis. Although this research orientation makes it possible to gain knowledge on such macro–micro dynamics, there remain uncertainties as to the exact mechanisms and consequences of these dynamics, particularly as they vary between different contexts.

Reflecting clients' responsibilities

Regarding clients' "transformation of the self", responsibilisation is embedded in citizenship, self-management, recovery, resilience and empowerment discourses. All these discourses expect clients to become self-governing and goal-oriented: for instance, in monitoring symptoms and seeking help, managing care contacts, making plans, re-entering the community and taking care of personal, everyday matters. Individuals are expected to actively manage their own health and make responsible lifestyle choices. As was shown in Chapters 5 and 6, the clients at the margins of welfare services on the one hand present themselves as people who try to reach the ideal "responsible self", whilst on the other hand they resist such cultural expectations as impossible or unreasonable due to their ill-health, limited resources and abilities. When the clients draw on advanced liberal responsibilisation expectations, they express that they need to, and can, make the required life changes by themselves in order to be a full citizen and to re-enter the community. In contrast, when resisting the idea of the responsible self, they use "fatalistic talk" and "drifting talk" to indicate that there are no possibilities available to try to change things for the better. Resisting "the responsible self", or not achieving it, locates the clients as prime candidates for more coercive re-responsibilisation, rehabilitation and education projects. Clients also identify risks of failures in recovery and are aware of gaps between societal expectations and their actions: for them the gap is alternatively something that is possible to overcome, or something that they just have to accept and adjust to.

Our analysis of clients' responsibilities raises some critical questions. Is trying to overcome the gap – to struggle to become more self-governed and active in the community – too demanding and risky for some clients? When does the principle of self-responsibility support clients' empowerment and change for the better, and when does it provide opportunities for blaming, abandonment, exclusion, exhaustion and disempowering defeats in their everyday lives? There are causal accounts that explain and demonstrate the difficulties in being a responsible self (see Chapter 5). However, relevant questions for the clients remain. What are legitimate accounts, excuses or justifications for not taking responsibility? What are sufficient activities for active citizens? This book stresses that the clients are active in making their way to better well-being and participation. However, to be active requires future prospects, support and resources, and is often accomplished partially and begrudgingly and carried out in gradual steps.

The situations and conditions in people's life courses can change rapidly, and we thus need to consider how the responsible self and irresponsible self are both legitimate and valued. There are times when we are able to care for ourselves and others, whilst at other times we are powerless, helpless and in need of others to take responsibility and to ensure our health and safety. Shifts in responsibilities may require a shorter or longer time, and more or less intensive support. To be active and responsible is made possible by offering resources and support (and control), and by strengthening reciprocal relations in the community. People usually want to be active, and have good reasons and justifications if they are not. Our studies on welfare practices demonstrate that workers understand these reasons and justifications and thus recognise the problems within the "big" discourse on self-responsibilisation, but they often are themselves caught "between a rock and a hard place" in encountering the clients and regulations.

Reflecting workers' responsibilities

In turn, welfare workers are also objects and subjects of responsibilisation, with conflicting discourses of managerialism, professional ethics, risk assessment and recovery. These discourses make workers personally accountable for the clients' engagement and commitment to services and progress, as well as for the economical sustainability of services. In other words, the grass-roots level workers are responsibilised by themselves, managers and commissioners to make the clients responsible for their conduct and recovery outcomes (see Chapters 8 and 9). We have demonstrated how the workers need to balance managerial expectations and clients' specific needs. Clients are not left to manage by themselves; instead, workers are busy planning, assessing, directing, controlling and coaching. Clients are expected to utilise professional advice and support. In turn, workers are expected to provide support for those who are entitled to services and included on their caseload. The workers are responsible for several issues, such as supporting clients in taking small risks and avoiding taking high risks, and in making appropriate use of services (see Chapters 7 and 8). In addition, the workers are responsible for managing the client flow and collaboration with other professionals in the field. This requires continual assessment of the clients' needs and what service they are entitled to; which client is to be transferred to which institution; and the scope of expertise and mandate of each professional in the network. This produces activity that aims to both limit and extend the workers' responsibilities in particular cases (see Chapter 9).

In the book, we have presented several technologies and techniques by which welfare workers carry out their various responsibilities at the institutional, collaborative and individual client levels. Institutional-level technologies include, for example, commissioning contracts, case-planning meetings, institutional forms and performance measures (see Chapters 7, 8 and 10). At the collaborative level, special discursive techniques were identified to distribute responsibilities between "us" and other workers involved with the client; this was summarised as exclusionary and inclusionary boundary work (see Chapter 9). The workers also use various discursive techniques to promote the clients' responsibilisation and to manage the distribution of responsibilities between themselves and the clients, such as planning, coaching, going along with, directing, giving advice and questioning the clients' willingness to change and their commitment to the service and recovery process (see Chapters 6, 7 and 8). These technologies and techniques demonstrate how responsibilisation is translated at the grass-roots level via particular artefacts, practices and discursive actions.

Political and practical implications

The purpose of the book is not to provide guidelines, to be a "toolkit" of how to advance or evaluate welfare practices: ethnomethodologically oriented research does not take as a starting point the question of whether stakeholders apply theories and policies in a "right" or "wrong", or "good" or "bad", manner. Rather, the interest is focused on more basic questions, such as how the discourses on governmentality and responsibilisation are oriented to and are put into practice by different ways of reasoning and acting. Stakeholders are considered to be active, reasonable people who act in the best possible way given their context and available knowledge. It is for them to judge what is a good or bad practice of responsibilisation. They also possess valuable knowledge that ought not to be bypassed in policy-level development work. The book makes the clients' and workers' practices and formulations visible and available to be used in developing policies and practices.

In turn, it is the researchers' task to make sense of and conceptualise the discourses and practices in play, and to demonstrate how different macro-level theories and policies might set up contradictions in real-life situations and produce conflicting, unexpected and unwanted consequences. As we have demonstrated, advanced liberal ways of understanding responsibilisation are occasionally present in the clients' and the workers' talk and actions at the margins of welfare; they also influence the ways strong welfare discourses – participation, empowerment, recovery, resilience, consumerism and personalisation – are interpreted in welfare encounters. For example, it is notable that welfare discourses and their key concepts can be "hijacked" for managerial and performance management purposes, sometimes in ways that distance the discourses from their more client-centred origins. However, responsibilisation is more complex and conflicting in practices at the margins of welfare services than the governmentality literature indicates. There are also competing discourses of responsibility, and alternatives to the advanced liberal way of responsibilisation. We have been discussing social, reciprocal, ethical and professional responsibilities that offer different ways to conceptualise responsibility and relations between different stakeholders in society. So, there is often also room for professional interpretation and discretion.

It seems that realising responsibilisation leads easily to pressing ethical contradictions. We have located various dilemmas and practical difficulties which the clients and the workers face when responsibilisation expectations clash with alternative professional theories and ethics, and with individual clients' complex situations and everyday problems. In order to produce adequate practices and client outcomes, it needs to be considered when, where and to whom responsibilisation is a good fit, and whether there are more suitable discourses to settle the relations (responsibilities and rights) between citizens, clients, welfare workers, institutions and the state. This kind of evaluation is continuously accomplished by grass-roots level actors at the margins of welfare by challenging and resisting responsibilisation expectations for justifiable reasons. For example, in some situations, providing intensive care for, or giving direction to, a vulnerable client might be more appropriate and effective than strong responsibilisation measures.

We perceived that managing responsibilities is very much about managing conflicting expectations, interests, uncertainties and sensitive matters in changing interactional contexts. This "messiness" of everyday practices needs to be captured, understood and appreciated when constructing future welfare policies and practices. There are creative and empowering ways to put responsibilisation into practice that are beneficial for workers' and clients' performance, such as coaching and risk assessment. However, in some circumstances, the very same techniques may produce disempowering results; for example, the client may perceive more clearly his/her deficiencies, which thereby strengthens self-stigmatisation and isolation. Thus applying responsibilisation needs to be accompanied by ethical and professional judgement and reflection. There is the risk that too much responsibility, for a client with limited resources, abilities and choices, may result in disempowering outcomes. At the margins of welfare services, responsibility is not just an individualistic and consumerist phenomenon, but is rather a reciprocal, social and negotiable construction embedded in being human. It is negotiated in relation to choices, risks, resources and other people and is thus a collective and societal accomplishment. Accordingly, there are many ways to be a responsible self.

References

Garfinkel, H. (1967) *Studies in Ethnomethodology*, Cambridge: Polity Press.
Rose, N. (1990) *Governing the Soul: The shaping of the private self*, London: Routledge.

Index

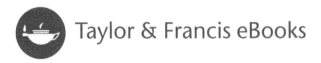

Taylor & Francis eBooks

Helping you to choose the right eBooks for your Library

Add Routledge titles to your library's digital collection today. Taylor and Francis ebooks contains over 50,000 titles in the Humanities, Social Sciences, Behavioural Sciences, Built Environment and Law.

Choose from a range of subject packages or create your own!

Benefits for you

- » Free MARC records
- » COUNTER-compliant usage statistics
- » Flexible purchase and pricing options
- » All titles DRM-free.

REQUEST YOUR **FREE** INSTITUTIONAL TRIAL TODAY

Free Trials Available
We offer free trials to qualifying academic, corporate and government customers.

Benefits for your user

- » Off-site, anytime access via Athens or referring URL
- » Print or copy pages or chapters
- » Full content search
- » Bookmark, highlight and annotate text
- » Access to thousands of pages of quality research at the click of a button.

eCollections – Choose from over 30 subject eCollections, including:

Archaeology	Language Learning
Architecture	Law
Asian Studies	Literature
Business & Management	Media & Communication
Classical Studies	Middle East Studies
Construction	Music
Creative & Media Arts	Philosophy
Criminology & Criminal Justice	Planning
Economics	Politics
Education	Psychology & Mental Health
Energy	Religion
Engineering	Security
English Language & Linguistics	Social Work
Environment & Sustainability	Sociology
Geography	Sport
Health Studies	Theatre & Performance
History	Tourism, Hospitality & Events

For more information, pricing enquiries or to order a free trial, please contact your local sales team:
www.tandfebooks.com/page/sales

The home of
Routledge books

www.tandfebooks.com

For Product Safety Concerns and Information please contact our EU
representative GPSR@taylorandfrancis.com
Taylor & Francis Verlag GmbH, Kaufingerstraße 24, 80331 München, Germany